European School of Oncology

Monographs

Series Editor: U. Veronesi

The European School of Oncology gratefully acknowledges sponsorship for the Task Force received from

ZENECA Pharmaceuticals

A. Howell (Ed.)

Endocrine Therapy of Breast Cancer VI

With 33 Figures and 20 Tables

Springer-Verlag
Berlin Heidelberg New York
London Paris Tokyo
Hong Kong Barcelona
Budapest

Anthony Howell, M.D., FRCP
CRC Department of Medical Oncology
University of Manchester
Christie Hospital NHS Trust
Wilmslow Road
Manchester M20 9BX, U.K.

ISBN-13:978-3-642-78816-1 e-ISBN-13:978-3-642-78814-7
DOI: 10.1007/978-3-642-78814-7

Library of Congress Cataloging-in-Publication Data
Endocrine therapy of breast cancer VI / A. Howell, ed.
(Monographs / European School of Oncology)
Includes bibliographical references.
ISBN-13:978-3-642-78816-1

1. Breast--Cancer--Immunotherapy. 2. Estrogen--Antagonists--Therapeutic use. I. Howell, A. (Anthony) II. Series: Monographs (European School of Oncology) [DNLM: 1. Breast Neoplasms--drug therapy. 2. Hormones--therapeutic use. WP 870 E55558 1994] RC280.B8E525 1994 616.99'449061--dc20 DNLM/DLC for Library of Congress

Softcover reprint of the hardcover 1st edition 1994

Typesetting: Camera ready by editor

19/3130 - 5 4 3 2 1 0 — Printed on acid-free paper

Foreword

The European School of Oncology came into existence to respond to a need for information, education and training in the field of the diagnosis and treatment of cancer. There are two main reasons why such an initiative was considered necessary. Firstly, the teaching of oncology requires a rigorously multidisciplinary approach which is difficult for the Universities to put into practice since their system is mainly disciplinary orientated. Secondly, the rate of technological development that impinges on the diagnosis and treatment of cancer has been so rapid that it is not an easy task for medical faculties to adapt their curricula flexibly.

With its residential courses for organ pathologies and the seminars on new techniques (laser, monoclonal antibodies, imaging techniques etc.) or on the principal therapeutic controversies (conservative or mutilating surgery, primary or adjuvant chemotherapy, radiotherapy alone or integrated), it is the ambition of the European School of Oncology to fill a cultural and scientific gap and, thereby, create a bridge between the University and Industry and between these two and daily medical practice.

One of the more recent initiatives of ESO has been the institution of permanent study groups, also called task forces, where a limited number of leading experts are invited to meet once a year with the aim of defining the state of the art and possibly reaching a consensus on future developments in specific fields of oncology.

The ESO Monograph series was designed with the specific purpose of disseminating the results of these study group meetings, and providing concise and updated reviews of the topic discussed.

It was decided to keep the layout relatively simple, in order to restrict the costs and make the monographs available in the shortest possible time, thus overcoming a common problem in medical literature: that of the material being outdated even before publication.

Umberto Veronesi
Chairman Scientific Committee
European School of Oncology

Foreword

Contents

Introduction

Anthony Howell

Department of Medical Oncology, Christie Hospital, Wilmslow Road, Manchester M20 9BX, United Kingdom

The aim of the Breast Cancer Task Force of the European School of Oncology is to bring together in one volume some of the newer developments in our understanding and treatment of breast cancer for clinicians and interested laboratory workers. One of the delights and also one of the difficulties for those with an interest in this disease, is that it involves such a wide span of subjects from molecular biology to terminal care. Review articles help us to keep abreast of such a broad field. The contributions in this volume reflect the breadth of the subject and we hope they will be of interest.

An additional aim of the series is to bridge the gap between the laboratory and the clinic. To this end more than half of the contributors are laboratory scientists who have an excellent grasp of the clinical problem. The remainder of the contributors are clinicians with laboratory interests. Three chapters are on new approaches to therapy using pure antioestrogens (Wakeling), antiprogestins (Klijn) and a novel form of immunotherapy (Taylor-Papadimitriou) which represent interesting approaches already in clinical trial. It is likely that new therapies will evolve from a greater understanding of growth control mechanisms of breast cancer cells and recent knowledge in this area is summarized by Sutherland and his colleagues. The antioestrogens represent the major form of endocrine therapy in use now; however, nearly all patients become resistant to therapy and insights (given here by Parker and by Jordan) into the mechanism of resistance may help us find ways to circumvent it.

There is now intense interest in assessment of risk in, and prevention of, breast cancer. Bishop gives a comprehensive review of the new genetics of breast cancer, indicating how close we are to prediction. Such is the rate of progress in this area that it is likely that the BRCAI breast cancer gene will have been cloned by the time this monograph is published. Also, tamoxifen prevention trials will be well under way. New approaches to prevention will almost certainly come from greater understanding of the normal breast in the early events in the neoplastic process and these are summarized by Howell and colleagues. Finally, Kaufmann highlights the problem of the deficiencies in our knowledge of the interaction between endocrine and chemotherapy for early breast cancer, and Coates gives a masterly review of recent developments in the assessment of quality of life.

Recent Progress in Breast Cancer Genetic Epidemiology

D. Timothy Bishop[1], Nancy Eby [2] and Jenny Chang-Claude [2]

1 ICRF Genetic Epidemiology Laboratory, Ashley Wing, St. James's University Hospital, Beckett Street, Leeds LS9 7TF, United Kingdom
2 Division of Epidemiology, German Cancer Research Centre, Im Neuenheimer Feld 280, 6900 Heidelberg, Germany

The large number of analytical studies of breast cancer epidemiology have identified a variety of risk factors; among these one of the most consistently reported is the previous occurrence of breast cancer in a close female relative (for reviews see [1] and [2]). The observation of the importance of family history is not novel in that many diseases including most cancers [3,4] have a positive family history as a risk factor, and at least for the common cancers, the strength of the association is similar to that observed for breast cancer. The relative risk associated with a family history is of the order of 2 to 3, although, as will be discussed later, the precise magnitude depends on a number of factors including the age of onset in the index case. The difficulty with such an observation is that in itself it does not indicate the nature of the true underlying risk factors which could be genetic or environmental with members of the same family being more similar in their exposure to the environmental risk factors.
The evidence that genes contribute to risk comes from the observation of a number of extensive pedigrees which are clearly segregating a rare autosomal dominant gene for susceptibility as seen in the example in Figure 1. In these families, carriers of the breast cancer susceptibility pass on the susceptibility to half their children on average. Males as well as females can carry the susceptibility gene although few (if any) males themselves develop breast cancer. Women who are genetically susceptible are at dramatically increased risk of breast cancer and have a lifetime risk that approaches certainty for developing breast cancer. One of the first documentations of such families is the report in the nineteenth century by the neurologist Paul Broca, of his wife's family; in that family, 10 of the 24 women had died of breast cancer [5]. In more recent times, among many other reports, several authors have documented large numbers of families [6, 7 and refs. contained therein, 8 and refs. contained therein, 9]. These reports are, of course, anecdotal but provide convincing evidence of dominant inheritance of breast cancer in a small number of families. Additional evidence of genetic aetiology is the increased occurrence of breast cancer in other genetic and familial cancer syndromes such as the Li-Fraumeni syndrome which is characterised by an autosomal dominant pattern of diverse neoplasms in children and young adults with a predominance of breast cancer, soft tissue sarcomas, osteosarcoma, and excesses of brain tumours, adrenocortical carcinomas and leukaemia [10,11].
Since the simple dichotomy of a positive family history (yes/no) is so crude, many recent studies have examined the precise genetic relationship of affected relatives to cases. From this information and the age, sex and genetic relationship of the unaffected relatives, a more detailed examination of family aggregation can be performed. There are several consistent conclusions to these analyses; primarily among these is that mothers and sisters of cases have a qualitatively similar risk of breast cancer and that this risk is elevated over the general population. A statistical technique termed "segregation analysis" allows the comparison of various models as explanations of the pattern of aggregation of disease in families. These analyses have almost all suggested that breast cancer susceptibility is inherited in some families as an autosomal dominant with partial penetrance, that is, not all female gene carriers develop breast cancer.

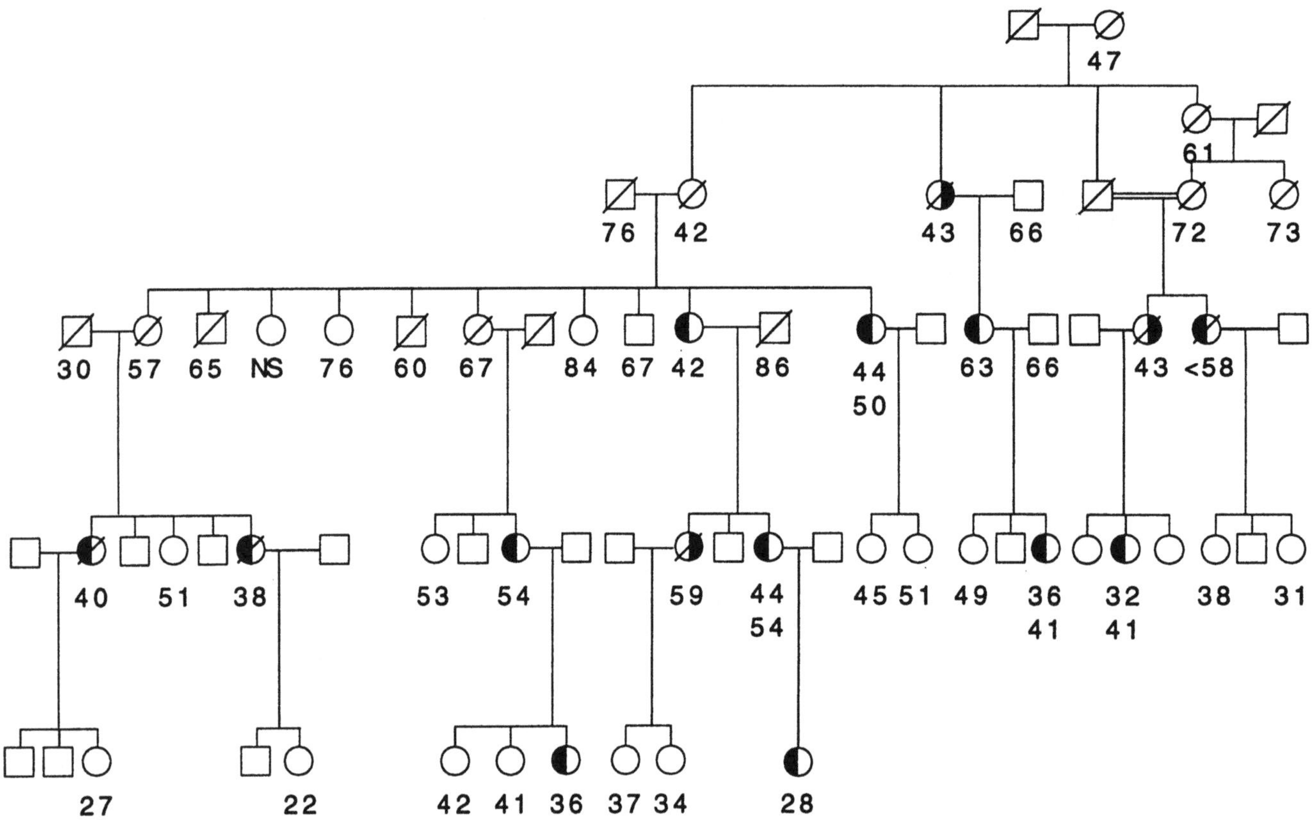

Fig. 1. A large breast-ovarian cancer family studied in Leeds, England. The breast cancer cases have the left side of the symbol shaded while the ovarian cancer cases have the right side of the symbol shaded. The age at diagnosis of the cancers is given below each affected woman. Some women have had two cancers and both of these ages of diagnosis are given under the symbol.

While segregation analysis can suggest the involvement of an important gene, the definitive conclusion of such a gene can only be made when this gene has been mapped. We say that such a gene has been mapped when its location on one of the 22 autosomal chromosomes is known.

In 1990, Dr Mary-Claire King and colleagues [12] reported the mapping of a breast cancer susceptibility gene to human chromosome 17q; this gene has been labelled "BRCA1". Subsequent studies have confirmed the importance of BRCA1 [13] in a subset of families; this subset includes a substantial proportion of large, early-onset families. However, BRCA1 appears to play only a minor role in family aggregation of breast cancer overall since linkage is not observed in a large number of small families.

In this review, we examine the role of genetic predisposition for breast cancer; there have been few studies of family history and postmenopausal breast cancer so this review deals almost exclusively with early onset breast cancer.

Epidemiological Studies

Epidemiological studies have consistently shown that a woman with a first-degree relative (mother, sister, or daughter) with breast cancer has an increased risk of breast cancer [1,14]. To quantify the risk associated with a family history of breast cancer, some studies have reported risk relative to the general population (relative risk) while others have reported results from lifetable analyses (cumulative lifetime risk). The major factors that have been examined in recent studies are (i) the effect of tumour laterality in the index case on familial risk, (ii) the variation in family risk with age of onset of the index case and (iii) the variation in

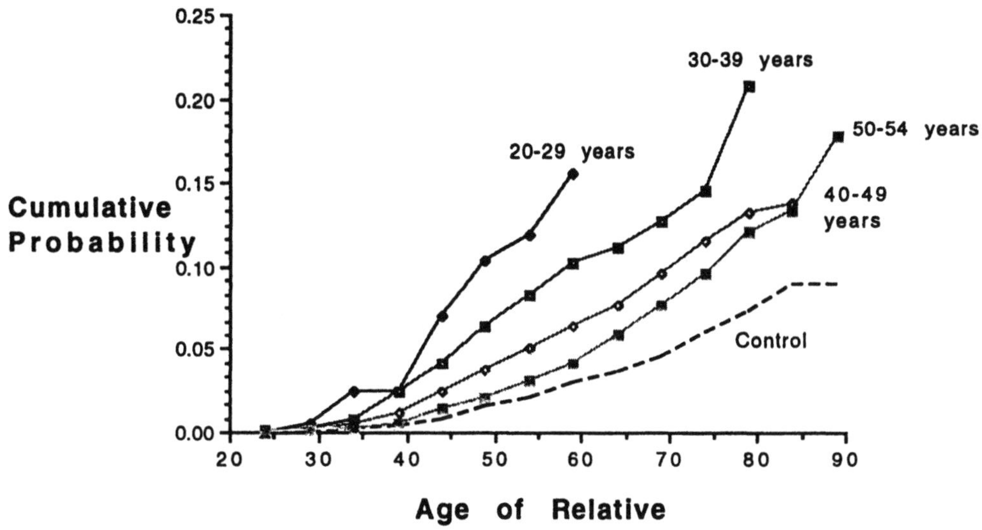

Fig. 2. The cumulative probability of breast cancer by age for female first-degree relatives of breast cancer cases by the age of onset of the case as well as the corresponding probability for controls for comparison purposes. Similar figures are given in [19]; the numbers used to draw these figures were provided by Dr. Elizabeth Claus [19].

risk with the number of cases already observed in the family. These questions are to some extent motivated by the observation that premenopausal breast cancer, in particular, may have a stronger genetic aetiology since a family history of breast cancer [14] and a greater tendency to bilateral occurrence [15] are more common in this group of cases.

The two largest epidemiological studies involving family history conducted to date are the Breast Cancer Detection and Demonstration Project (BCDDP) study [16,17] and the Cancer and Steroid Hormone Study (CASH) [18-20]. Many other studies have evaluated family history as a risk factor but have been limited by their sample sizes so we focus attention on these two studies. The CASH study is a population based study of 4730 breast cancer cases diagnosed before the age of 55 years and 4688 controls. In this study [19], the cumulative risk of breast cancer by age 59 was estimated to be 0.061 for mothers of cases as compared to 0.029 for mothers of controls and 0.065 for sisters of cases and 0.029 for sisters of controls. Overall, the risk for mothers of cases was twice that of mothers of controls and for sisters of cases the risk was 2.3 times the risk for sisters of controls.

Given that risks to mothers and sisters are similar it is useful to group these two together to estimate the absolute risk for first-degree relatives of cases. Figure 2 shows the cumulative risk of breast cancer in first degree relatives of cases by the age at diagnosis of the case. At all ages the relatives show an increased risk over controls and this risk is greater when the age at onset of the case is the youngest. Having an additional first-degree relative (mother or sister) affected with breast cancer (Fig. 3), further increases a woman's risk. On the basis of hazard analysis [19], sisters with affected mothers had an estimated 3.9-fold increased risk over sisters whose mother was unaffected.

Byrne and colleagues [17] in their analysis of 2908 breast cancer cases and 3180 controls from the BCDDP in the United States, found that a maternal history of breast cancer increased the risk of breast cancer at any age (RR = 1.9 overall); a sister with breast cancer produced an overall relative risk of 2.3. A maternal history of breast cancer had the same approximately 2-fold effect on risk of breast cancer at all ages. However, an affected sister increased the risk 7-fold for breast cancer before age 45 years, while the risk was reduced to only 2-fold for onset after age 50 years. Moreover, diagnosis under 50 years of age not only increased the risk in sisters, it also increased their risk of developing the disease at a younger age.

A few studies have looked at the risk in families of cases with bilateral disease. Ottman and colleagues [21] in a population-based series of bilateral cases found an increased risk of breast cancer in sisters (RR = 5.5 for cases diagnosed before the age of 50 years). These results are consistent with those from the BCDDP which found a relative risk (RR) of 4.7 for sisters of bilateral cases. The CASH study

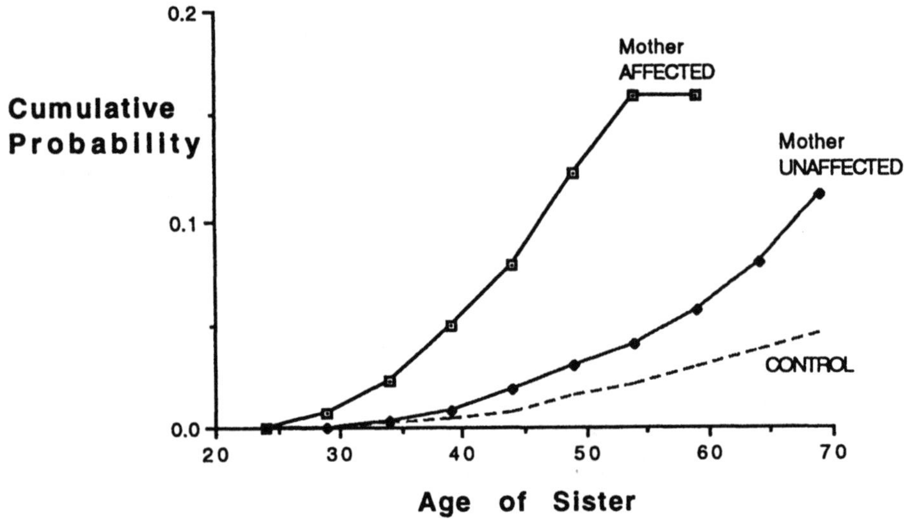

Fig. 3. The cumulative probability of breast cancer by age for sisters of breast cancer cases depending on the disease status of the mother of the case as well as the cumulative probability for controls for comparison purposes. Similar figures are given in [19]; the numbers used to draw these figures were provided by Dr. Elizabeth Claus [19].

did not report risk to mothers because of suggested underreporting of breast cancer in mothers of controls [19]. However, the BCDDP study [17] found a RR of 1.9 for mothers of bilateral cases suggesting that these mothers are also at increased risk but their risk is somewhat lower than that for sisters. Because of the design of the CASH study, there was not a representative sample of subjects to examine the families of bilateral cases.

Family history of breast cancer as a risk factor does not appear to be confounded by other breast cancer risk factors [17,22]. While some of the other risk factors for breast cancer such as age at menarche and age at menopause may themselves be genetically determined, controlling for these factors appears not to alter the risk associated with family history [17]. Thus, familial clustering of breast cancer does not appear to be measuring familial aggregation of these other risk factors. Results from several studies suggest that age at menarche [17,22], age at first live birth [17,26], benign breast disease [27], long-term oral contraceptive use, and age at menopause [17,22] may modify the effect of family history on breast cancer risk. Among these risk factors, age at menarche and age at first live birth have been found to be stronger risk factors for premenopausal disease than postmenopausal disease.

Segregation Analysis

The epidemiological studies have essentially all documented that relatives of breast cancer patients are at increased risk of breast cancer (see above). Many of these studies are population based and show systematic ascertainment of a consecutive series of cases. Until recently, studies of the genetics of susceptibility to breast cancer have not been systematically pursued and, instead, the literature consists of a number of reports of anecdotal families with clear evidence of dominantly inherited susceptibility with onset being at particularly early ages. One of the first such reports is by Broca who documented the family history of his wife [5]. Subsequently, Dr. Eldon Gardner reported on a Utah family initially ascertained because of breast cancer in 3 close relatives [28] but shown after some extensive work to be part of a large kindred. Gardner and colleagues reported approximately every decade on the continuing story of increased incidence of breast cancer in this family [29-31]. At the time of the last report, 29 cases of breast cancer had been documented in this family [31]. Similar reports have been produced by many others, including Dr. Henry Lynch and his colleagues in Omaha, Nebraska [7 and refs. contained therein] and Dr. David Anderson and colleagues in Houston, Texas [9 and refs. contained therein]. Each of these authors document dominantly inherited susceptibility to early-onset breast cancer.

Segregation analysis is a statistical technique which assesses the extent of family aggregation and attempts to relate this aggregation to underlying mechanisms [32]. Basically, from the distribution of the number of affected children in families among the various combinations of the parental disease states, segregation analysis examines the most plausible explanations of this distribution from the models formulated. Segregation analysis is most informative in carefully identified, population-based studies in which at least the disease state of the first and second-degree relatives of the cases has been determined. However, practicalities such as the difficulties of obtaining medical records on second-degree relatives often preclude such extensions and so many studies relate only to the parents, siblings and offspring of cases. This review concentrates on 3 large systematic population-based studies reported to date. There have been numerous other studies which have performed segregation analysis on small numbers of families usually ascertained in an ad hoc fashion and usually under the assumption that breast cancer is determined as an autosomal dominant gene. Because these studies do not relate to the general population, they are excluded from this review, although it is fair to indicate that to a large extent their conclusions have been similar to the population-based series.

The models that have been considered to explain the family aggregation of breast cancer have included (i) models in which a single gene is assumed to be responsible for the family aggregation (the "major gene model"); (ii) models in which multiple genes each with small but similar effects ("polygenes") are important (the "multifactorial model"); (iii) a model in which both major genes and polygenes are relevant and supplement the effect of each other (the "mixed model"), and (iv) a model in which family aggregation of disease is entirely due to an unmeasured environmental factor shared by members of the family (the "environmental model").

The 3 largest systematic population-based studies are the 200 families collected by Jacobsen [6], the 254 nuclear families collected by Dr. Joan Slack and colleagues [33], and the CASH study (1579 nuclear families reported in [34], and 4730 nuclear families including those reported in [34] which were analysed in [20]).

In 1946, Jacobsen reported on the family histories of cases taken from a sequential series approximately two-thirds of whom yielded family information on first and second-degree relatives [6]. Williams and Anderson [35] performed segregation analysis of these families under the mixed model and found evidence of a rare dominant gene with no evidence of any residual polygenic heritability, that is, that once a major gene was asserted there was no evidence that polygenes played any further role. Iselius and colleagues reanalysed these same families and changed various technical assumptions regarding the modelling of the mode of inheritance [36]; these assumptions relate to the changing proportions of susceptible women in the general population at older ages as those genetically susceptible are on average affected at a younger age and some will die at a young age of breast cancer. The approach of [36] is an approximation that, intuitively at least, should improve the test of the fit of the model to the data. Although their analysis shows less evidence for a major gene than did the Williams and Anderson [35] analysis, the same qualitative conclusion applied concerning the mode of inheritance. Some of the quantitative predictions obtained from the two methods of analysis do, however, differ. Iselius and colleagues [36] estimated that the at birth frequency of carriers was commoner than predicted by Williams and Anderson [35] (1.8% of women vs. 1.5%) and that the lifetime penetrance for breast cancer for women carrying the genetic susceptibility was 0.78 as compared to the estimate of 0.57 [35]. In terms of population estimates, Iselius and colleagues [36] estimated that 73% of cases diagnosed between the ages of 30 and 39 years would be gene carriers as compared to 62% in the initial analysis [35].

The British study by Iselius and colleagues [35] consisted of the families of 254 cases not selected for family history but 50 of whom were selected on the basis of age of onset, and 416 families collected on the basis of family history alone. Again this study suggested that breast cancer susceptibility was inherited as a rare autosomal dominant gene in some families. The analysis of the two sets of families gave considerably different results but the two sets of results were not significantly different because of the poor resolution of the former set of families. For instance, the analysis of the families selected on the basis of family history suggested that at birth 0.4% of women were genetically susceptible while the other series suggested that 5.6% of women were susceptible but with a correspondingly lower lifetime risk. The best estimate of all families combined was that 0.6% of women were susceptible and that the lifetime risk for breast cancer in carriers was 0.83. Forty percent of cases diagnosed between the ages of 30 and 39 years were estimated to be due to this gene. This latter figure is considerably lower than those estimated from the Danish pedigrees discussed above although the lifetime risks for carriers are similar.

Claus and colleagues [20] performed segregation analysis on the CASH families and again showed that a rare dominant gene without any residual polygenic heritability best explained the family aggregation. This study estimated that the lifetime risk for breast cancer in susceptible women was essentially certain and that at birth on average 0.66% of women carried the susceptibility. Under the best fitting model, approximately 40% of cases diagnosed in the general population between the ages of 30 and 39 years appeared to be due to this gene.

Linkage Analysis

The results from the segregation analyses suggest that breast cancer is inherited through an autosomal dominant gene in some families. The standard method for identifying the locations of such genes is through "linkage analysis" [37]. In this approach, family members are typed for a number of DNA markers, each of which has a known genetic location. Markers are defined by a DNA sequence which shows variation among the general population; these variants are called "alleles". To be as informative as possible, these markers must show large numbers of alleles, none of which is common in the general population (that is, less than 25% of the general population should carry each variant) and each marker must be accessible to routine assay. Basically with this approach, since there are so many alleles, the parental origin of each allele identified in the child can usually be identified; suppose for instance the father of a child has the two alleles 1 and 2 while the mother has variants 3 and 4 and their child has the alleles 1 and 3, then the 1 allele must have been inherited from the child's father and the 3 allele from the child's mother. If, within a family with breast cancer susceptibility, a specific allele from this marker is usually inherited together with the breast cancer susceptibility, then we say that the susceptibility is linked to this marker (Fig. 4).

Linkage implies that the susceptibility gene and the DNA marker must lie in close proximity to each other and hence knowledge of the chromosomal position of the marker allows us to identify the chromosomal region where the susceptibility gene must lie. "Linkage analysis" involves the examination of various genetic polymorphisms with known chromosomal loca-

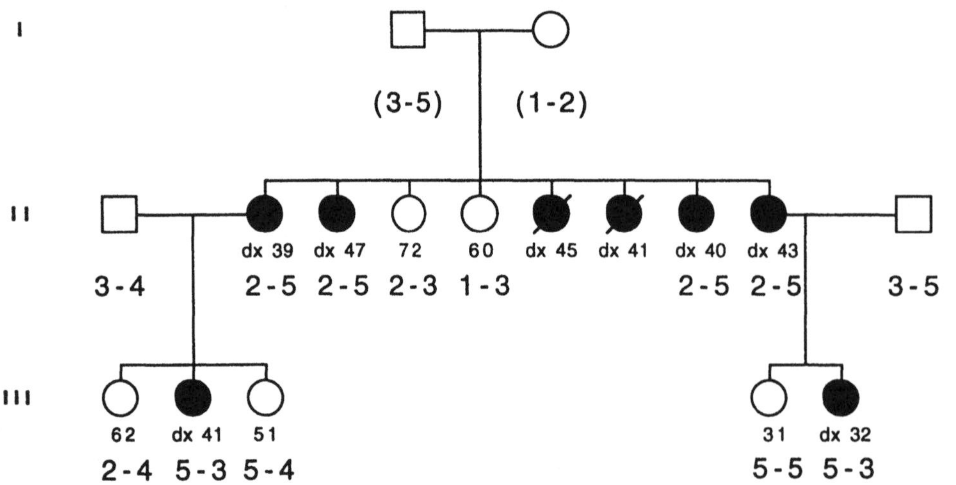

Fig. 4. A family from [39] showing linkage to a DNA marker on chromosome 17q. The age of onset of affected women is given under each pedigree symbol (dx <age of onset>) as is the current age for unaffected women. Each person who provided a DNA sample has been typed for the DNA marker and the two recognised alleles are shown under the age for each person. The grandparents at the top of the pedigree did not provide DNA samples but we can infer from the pedigree structure that one grandparent has the alleles 3 and 5 while the other has the alleles 1 and 2. In fact, for visual simplicity, we have assumed that the grandfather had the former combination of alleles. Within the family, the breast cancer gene is inherited together with the 5 allele from the marker locus. Each person in the family who has inherited the 5 allele from the grandfather has developed breast cancer at a young age except for two women in the third generation who by implication are at high risk of carrying the breast cancer gene (one is unaffected at age 51 while the other is unaffected at age 31).

tions in selected pedigrees until one of them is shown to be linked to the susceptibility gene. The consistency of the joint transmission within families is an indication as to the precise distance between the gene and the marker since large segments of chromosome will only sometimes be inherited intact by a child from the parent while shorter segments will more often be inherited intact; the more consistent the transmission, the closer the two locations are to each other.

Until the 1980s, when large numbers of polymorphic DNA markers regularly spaced throughout the human genome started to become available, phenotypic markers of blood groups, blood enzymes, and serum proteins were used for linkage analyses. Weak evidence for linkage was suggested for the ABO-blood group, properdin factor B, glutamate-pyruvate transaminase, Rhesus blood group and esterase D, but under the assumption that all families were due to the same gene, these findings were not confirmed in other pedigree studies. This assumption is now known to be incorrect since breast cancer has been shown to be genetically heterogeneous (see below), so that it is still plausible that other breast cancer genes could lie close to these markers. Subsequently, 8 oncogenes (H-ras, K-ras, N-ras, myc, myb, erb A-2, int-2, RAF1) were ruled out due to the lack of close linkage to breast cancer susceptibility in 12 families with 87 breast cancer cases [38].

Based on reports of DNA amplification within the chromosome 17q region in breast tumours and the knowledge that several genes related to normal breast development and breast cancer map to this area, Dr. Mary-Claire King and colleagues [39] investigated and provided evidence for close linkage of a breast cancer gene with a marker called D17S74 on 17q12-q21; this gene has been labelled "BRCA1" [13]. The linkage was confined to those families with average age of onset less than 45 years. Confirmation through replication in other families was described in [40]. In their study, 3 out of 5 families (60%) were shown to be due to BRCA1. These families were breast-ovarian families in that some obligate gene carriers developed ovarian cancer while others developed breast cancer.

The Cancer Family Study Group Breast Cancer Linkage Consortium, a group of European and American investigators, typed 6 markers on chromosome 17q, spanning the plausible region for BRCA1 around D17S74 in 214 breast cancer families. Fifty-seven of the families contained at least one case of ovarian cancer (these families are termed "breast-ovarian" families) while the remaining 157 contained only cases of breast cancer ("breast cancer only" families). The Consortium confirmed the previously published linkage and then were able to discuss various issues related to the genetic epidemiology of breast cancer [41].

A major issue that can be addressed when linked markers have been identified in some families is the issue of genetic heterogeneity. Since there was evidence that some families were due to BRCA1 while others were not, the natural question to ask is whether there are clinical features that distinguish these two types of families. In the Consortium results, there was a clear difference between the "breast-ovarian" cancer families and the families with breast cancer cases only with respect to genetic heterogeneity. Overall, the proportion of linked families was estimated to be 62%. However, all 57 "breast-ovarian" families were consistent with linkage while only 45% of the "breast cancer only" families showed linkage. The genetic heterogeneity observed in "breast cancer only" families appears to be age-dependent, with an estimated 67% of families with an average age of onset before 45 being linked compared to 19% of families with mean onset between 45 and 55 years, and 38% for families with average onset after age 55. The probability of linkage in these families also appears to be related to the number of breast cancer cases. The highest proportion of linked families (72%) was found amongst families with 5 or more cases of breast cancer diagnosed before the age of 45 years.

In "breast cancer only" families with 3 or less cases in total, there was little evidence of linkage [41]. There were also only a few large families which did not appear compatible with linkage. Taken together, these data suggest that the BRCA1 gene may be responsible for breast cancer in families with 4 or more cases in the general population. The majority of the genetic expression of breast cancer, however, may not be explained by BRCA1 and other breast cancer susceptibility genes may be important in those families. A second issue that can be addressed when linked markers are available is the estimation of the actual risk of cancer in carriers of the breast cancer gene. The penetrance of BRCA1 was estimated in "breast-ovarian" families and apparently linked "breast cancer only" families to be 59% by age 50 and 82% by age 70. When the two types of families were considered separately, the estimated penetrances were 67% by age 50 and 76% by age 70 in the "breast-ovary" families and 49% by age 50 and 90% by age 70 in the "breast cancer only" families; these two sets of estimates are not significantly different from each other.

While the Consortium analysis could not provide detailed information about the location of BRCA1 on 17q, various other observations have been made to narrow the region that must contain BRCA1. The current "best" region is between the DNA marker D17S183 and the gene for the thyroid hormone receptor alpha locus, THRA1, a region of perhaps 4,000,000 DNA base-pairs [42]; the rapid resolution of this region makes it likely that the DNA sequence of BRCA1 will soon be known.

Since BRCA1 does not explain all cases of inherited susceptibility to breast cancer, other genes have also been examined. The oestrogen receptor (ER) gene located on 6q24-q27 is regarded as a candidate susceptibility gene because of its biological activity in human breast cancer. Since postmenopausal breast tumours are more likely to be ER-positive, Zuppan and colleagues investigated linkage with this locus in 11 breast cancer families with late onset disease and found interesting but not conclusive evidence of linkage in one extended family [43]. The possibility of a susceptibility gene for late onset disease is enticing; however, the reported linkage results require confirmation in other families with late onset disease.

Mutations of the p53 gene has been identified in fibroblast DNA from members of 5 families with the Li-Fraumeni Syndrome in which a frequent occurrence of breast cancer has been observed [44]. It is possible that some breast cancer families will in fact be Li-Fraumeni families where the associated tumours have not yet appeared in the families.

Discussion

Genetic factors clearly contribute to risk of breast cancer since there are numerous families which show unequivocal evidence for a dominant gene or genes. The families that have been reported to date are largely families in which breast cancer occurs at an unusually young age; in fact, many of these families have an average age of onset for breast cancer of 45 years or less. In 1990, a report from Dr. Mary-Claire King's laboratory in Berkeley provided evidence that in some families a relevant gene (now called "BRCA1") was located on human chromosome 17q [39].

Subsequent reports culminating in the results from a collaborative study of 214 families have confirmed the finding and have made clearer the importance of this gene [41]. The major surprise of these studies was that all of the families which contained cases of both breast and ovarian cancer were consistent with being due to BRCA1 as were the majority of the families with 5 or more cases of breast cancer but without any cases of ovarian cancer. The majority of the breast-ovary families also contain more than 5 cases of breast cancer so the largest families (in terms of the number of breast cases) are mainly attributable to BRCA1.

Detailed analysis in these large families shows that BRCA1 lies in a well defined, small region of that chromosome. The distance between the two DNA markers which flank BRCA1 is estimated to be at most 4cM apart, which means that in only 4 meioses out of 100 is there a recombination event between these two markers [42]; the implication of this fact is that the examination of the inheritance of these markers in these BRCA1 families can be used to predict which women in the families have the inherited susceptibility to breast cancer. Clinically these or equivalent markers could be used to offer the option of carrier status determination to women within the families, so that a woman who was initially at 50% risk of carrying the gene because the woman's mother is a gene carrier could be advised that either her risk of being a carrier is close to 100% or that it is essentially 0%, in which case the woman's risk is that of the general population. There is no experience with this opportunity to date and so it is not known what proportion of women in these families will choose to know this information.

In a clinical setting, only a small percentage of families reported because of a family history of 5 or more cases of breast cancer. The majority of families will contain 3 or less cases and in these types of families the role of BRCA1 is much more difficult to evaluate. In families with 3 or less cases of breast cancer diagnosed before the age of 60 years, there is no evidence that BRCA1 plays any significant role; of course some of these smaller families may be in fact subsets of these larger BRCA1 families but the implication is that this percentage is so low that the effect of BRCA1 is undetectable. The conclusion must therefore be that BRCA1 is important in those few high-risk, multiple case families but overall BRCA1 only explains a trivial portion of familial breast cancer. The majority of the family aggregations must therefore be due to other causes, perhaps other lower penetrance genes or perhaps exposure within families to environmentally determined risk factors. How important then are genes in the aetiology of breast cancer? While this round of progress really has not shed any light on the answer to this question, BRCA1 is important only in those families in which we always knew that genes were important; we must await further progress to be more definitive.

However, while the immediate clinical implications are relevant in only a few families, the importance of identifying this gene should not be underestimated. Potentially the most exciting feature of the knowledge is that we learn more about the aetiology of breast cancer overall either by understanding one of the genes in the progression to breast cancer or by understanding more about the environment in which tumours can develop. From the information on the linkage mapping, we know that there are various genes which are known to lie in the region and which are candidates for being the breast cancer gene. These candidates are: the gene for a truncated form of the human epidermal growth factor receptor, her2 (her2 is identical to erbB2 or neu), the gene for oestradiol-17ß dehydrogenase, the enzyme that catalyses the conversion of oestrone to oestradiol, the homebox 2 gene (HOX2), which plays a critical role in murine embryologic development, the gene for retinoic acid receptor (RARA), a protein that is a possible anticarcinogen, and the gene WNT3, the human counterpart of an integration site for the mouse mammary tumour virus [12]. However, if BRCA1 is not due to a mutation in one of these genes, we must search for other genes in that region. Current thinking in cancer genetics suggests that many "cancer genes" do not confer an elevated risk of cancer, rather they protect against cancer. Cancer only results when this gene is present in its damaged form (in this case by being inherited in a mutated, inactive form). Such genes are termed "tumour suppressor genes" (see, for instance, [45]). Of course, the vast majority of individuals will not have inherited mutations in this gene; however, damage can still occur somatically so that individual cells may lose the controlling effect of this gene. The evidence is accumulating that BRCA1 is such a tumour suppressor gene since one indication of such a status is that within breast cancer families due to BRCA1, breast tumours should have lost the "normal" version of BRCA1. A cancer gene now recognised to be a tumour suppressor gene is the APC gene (for a review see [46]). Inherited mutations in this gene lead to polyposis coli while the majority of colorectal carcinomas that arise outside the family setting have been shown to have damage to this particular gene (i.e., the changes have occurred somatically). In this example, mapping the gene for the rare polyposis syndrome families led to identifying a gene relevant in perhaps all colorectal carcinomas. This may be the situation for breast cancer, or maybe there are presently unrecognised processes at work. Only knowledge of this gene will tell us its role in breast cancer overall.

Acknowledgements

The authors would like to thank Dr. Elizabeth Claus for providing the numbers for Figures 2 and 3. Funding was provided by the British German Academic Collaboration Programme which is supported by the British Council and the Deutscher Akademischer Austauschdienst.

REFERENCES

1 Kelsey JL: A review of the epidemiology of human breast cancer. Epidemiol Rev 1979 (1):74-109
2 Petrakis NL, Ernster VL, King M-C: Breast. In: Schottenfeld D and Fraumeni JF Jr (eds) Cancer Epidemiology and Prevention. WB Saunders, Philadelphia 1982 pp 855-870
3 Cannon L, Bishop DT, Skolnick M, Hunt S, Lyon JL, Smart CR: Genetic epidemiology of prostate cancer in the Utah Mormon genealogy. Cancer Surveys 1982 (1):47-69
4 Cannon-Albright LA, Bishop DT, Goldgar C, Skolnick MH: Genetic predisposition to cancer. Important Adv Oncol 1989:39-55
5 Brocca PP: Trait des Tumeurs, Vols 1 and 2. P Asselin, Paris 1866-1869
6 Jacobsen O: Heredity in Breast Cancer; A Genetic and Clinical Study of Two Hundred Probands. Lewis, London 1946 pp 3-6
7 Lynch HT, Lynch JF: Genetics of common tumors. In: Lynch HT and Tautu P (eds) Recent Progress in the Genetic Epidemiology of Cancer. Springer Verlag, Heidelberg 1991 pp 3-17
8 Gardner EJ: Prevention and cure of hereditary cancers. In: Cairns J, Lyon JL, Skolnick M (eds) Banbury Report 4. Cancer Incidence in Defined Populations. Cold Spring Harbor Laboratory Press 1980 pp 365-377
9 Anderson DE: A genetic study of human breast cancer. JNCI 1972 (48):1029-1034
10 McKusick VA: Mendelian Inheritance in Man, 10th edition. Johns Hopkins University Press, Baltimore 1990
11 Li FP, Fraumeni JR Jr, Mulvihill JJ et al: A cancer family syndrome in twenty-four kindreds. Cancer Res 1988 (48):5358-5362
12 Hall JM, Lee MK, Newman B, Morrow JE, Anderson LA et al: Linkage of early-onset familial breast cancer to chromosome 17q21. Science 1990 (250):1684-1689
13 Solomon E, Ledbetter DH: Report of the committee on the genetic constitution of chromosome 17. Cytogenet Cell Genet 1991 (58):686-738
14 Anderson DE: Familial predisposition. In: Shottenfeld D and Fraumeni JF Jr (eds) Cancer Epidemiology and Prevention. WB Saunders, Philadelphia 1982 pp 483-493
15 Prior P, Waterhouse JAH: Incidence of bilateral tumours in a population-based series of breast cancer patients. I. Two approaches to an epidemiological analysis. Br J Cancer 1978 (37):620-634
16 Brinton LA, Williams RR, Hoover RN, Stegens NL, Feinleib M, Fraumeni JF Jr: Breast cancer risk factors among screening program participants. JNCI 1979 (62):37-43
17 Byrne C, Brinton LA, Haile RW, Schairer C: Heterogeneity of the effect of family history on breast cancer. Epidemiology 1991 (2):276-284
18 Sattin RW, Rubin GL, Webster LA, Huezo CM, Wingo P et al: Family history and the risk of breast cancer. JAMA 1985 (253):1908-1913
19 Claus EB, Risch NJ, Thompson WD: Age at onset as an indicator of familial risk of breast cancer. Am J Epidemiol 1990 (131):961-972
20 Claus EB, Risch N, Thompson WD: Genetic analysis of breast cancer in the Cancer and Steroid Hormone study. Am J Hum Genet 1991 (48):232-242
21 Ottman R, Pike MC, King MC, Casagrande JT, Henderson BE: Familial breast cancer in a population-based series. Am J Epidemiol 1986 (123):15-21
22 Bain C, Speizer FE, Rosner B, Belanger C, Hennekens CH: Family history of breast cancer as a risk factor for the disease. Am J Epidemiol 1980 (111):301-308
23 Tulinius H, Day NE, Bjarnason O, Geirsson G, Johannesson G et al: Familial breast cancer in Iceland. Int J Cancer 1982 (29):365-371
24 Tulinius H, Sigvaldason H, Oelafsdoettir G, Tryggvadoettir L: Epidemiology of breast cancer in families in Iceland. Am J Hum Genet (in press)
25 Brinton LA, Hoover R, Fraumeni JF Jr: Interaction of familial and hormonal risk factors for breast cancer. JNCI 1982 (69):817-822
26 Dupont WD, Page DL: Breast cancer risk associated with proliferative disease, age at first birth, and a family history of cancer. Am J Epidemiol 1987 (125):769-779
27 Page DL, Dupont WD: Anatomic markers of human premalignancy and risk of breast cancer. Cancer 1990 (66):1326-1335
28 Gardner EJ, Stephens FE: Breast cancer in one family group. Am J Hum Genet 1950 (2):30
29 Stephens FE, Gardner EJ, Woolf CM: A recheck of Kindred 107 which has shown a high frequency of breast cancer. Cancer 1958 (11):967
30 Gardner EJ: Thirty-year follow-up of a breast cancer kindred. Am J Hum Genet 1977 (29):45A
31 Bishop DT, Gardner EJ: Analysis of the genetic predisposition to cancer in individual pedigrees. In: Cairns J, Lyon JL, Skolnick M (eds) Banbury Report 4. Cancer Incidence in Defined Populations. Cold Spring Harbor Laboratory Press 1980 pp 389-408
32 Elston RC, Stewart J: A general model for the genetic analysis of pedigree data. Hum Heredit 1971 (21):523-541
33 Iselius L, Slack J, Littler M, Morton NE: Genetic epidemiology of breast cancer in Britain. Ann Hum Genet 1991 (55):151-159
34 Newman B, Austin MA, Lee M, King MC: Inheritance of human breast cancer: evidence for autosomal dominant transmission in high-risk families. Proc Natl Acad Sci 1988 (85):3044-3048
35 Williams WR, Anderson DE: Genetic epidemiology of breast cancer: segregation analysis of 200 Danish pedigrees. Genet Epidemiol 1984 (1):7-20
36 Iselius L, Littler M, Morton N: Transmission of breast cancer - a controversy resolved. Clin Genet 1992 (41):211-217
37 Ott J: Analysis of Human Genetic Linkage. The Johns Hopkins University Press, Baltimore and London 1985
38 Hall JM, Zuppan PJ, Anderson LA, Huey B, Carter C, King MC: Oncogenes and human breast cancer. Am J Hum Genet 1989 (44):577-584

39 Hall JM, Lee MK, Newman B, Morrow JE, Anderson LA et al: Linkage of early-onset familial breast cancer to chromosome 17q21. Science 1990 (250):1684-1689
40 Narod SA, Feunteun J, Lynch HT, Watson P, Conway T, Lynch J, Lenoir G: A familial breast-ovarian cancer locus on chromosome 17q21-q23. Lancet 1991 (2):82-83
41 Easton DF, Bishop DT, Ford D, Crockford GP: Genetic linkage analysis in familial breast and ovarian cancer - results from 214 families. To appear in Am J Hum Genet
42 Bowcock AM, Anderson LA, Black DM, Osborne-Lawrence S, Hall JM, Solomon E, King M-C: Polymorphisms in THRA1 and D17S181 flank a >4 cM interval for the breast-ovarian cancer gene on chromosome 17q. To appear in Am J Hum Genet
43 Zuppan P, Hall JM, Lee MK, Ponglikitmongkol M, King MC: Possible linkage of the estrogen receptor gene to breast cancer in a family with late-onset disease. Am J Hum Genet 1991 (48):1065-1068
44 Malkin D, Li FP, Strong LC, Fraumeni JF Jr, Nelson CE et al: Germ line p53 mutations in a familial syndrome of breast cancer, sarcomas, and other neoplasms. Science 1990 (9):555-578
46 Bishop DT, Thomas HFW: The genetics of colon cancer. Cancer Surveys 1990 (9):585-604

Hormonal Control of Breast Cancer Cell Cycle Progression

Robert L. Sutherland, Jenny A. Hamilton, Colin K.W. Watts and Elizabeth A. Musgrove

Cancer Biology Division, Garvan Institute of Medical Research, St Vincent's Hospital, Sydney, N.S.W. 2010, Australia

Detailed knowledge of the factors that control the proliferation and differentiation of normal and neoplastic breast epithelium, and the molecular basis of their action, is essential for a deeper understanding of the development and progression of human breast cancer. Identification of factors involved in growth regulation has been facilitated by studies on breast cancer cell lines representative of different tumour phenotypes which have provided important information on ligand-receptor interactions and signal transduction pathways [1]. These studies have been complemented by data on genetic abnormalities in human breast tumours which have identified candidate genes likely to contribute to the loss of normal growth control associated with tumourigenesis and disease progression [2].

The central role for oestrogenic sex steroids in the aetiology of breast cancer has long been recognised: evidence that oophorectomy could lead to regression of established tumours was first obtained last century. Later studies on carcinogen-induced mammary cancer demonstrated that oestrogen was essential for both the initiation and progression of mammary carcinoma [3]. These observations in association with later developments in the understanding of the structure and function of steroid hormone receptors ultimately led to the routine use of oestrogen receptor (ER) status as a marker of hormone-responsiveness and prognosis in breast cancer [4].

A further major development was the targeting of therapy via the ER with the clinical application of the synthetic nonsteroidal antioestrogen, tamoxifen. The subsequent widespread use of tamoxifen, first in advanced disease, then as adjuvant therapy and more recently as a preventive strategy for individuals at high risk of developing the disease, is undoubtedly one of the major advances in cancer therapy to occur during the past decade [5,6]. Tamoxifen therapy of breast cancer, however, is limited in two major ways. Only a proportion of tumours respond, presumably due to the absence of a functional ER system or loss of ER-mediated growth control, while initial responders often go on to develop resistance to the growth inhibitory effects of the antioestrogen [7]. Thus one of the immediate challenges in developing new therapeutic strategies for breast cancer is to identify other growth stimulatory and inhibitory molecules and to characterise the molecular basis of their action as modulators of growth and differentiation. Building on the experience with tamoxifen, the first receptor-targeted anticancer agent, researchers should feel confident that more detailed knowledge in this area will lead to further therapeutic advances. Indeed advances in experimental therapeutics targeted via the progesterone receptor [8], retinoic acid receptors [9], the epidermal growth factor receptor and c-*erb*B-2 [10] provide examples of exciting developments built upon such a strategy.

With an aim to identifying key regulatory factors for breast cancer cell proliferation this review summarises contemporary knowledge on factors that control rates of cell cycle progression in human breast cancer cells. The effects of these factors on the expression of genes thought to have roles in cell cycle control is summarised and has aided in identifying candidate key cell cycle regulatory genes.

Hormone and Growth Factor Regulation of Breast Cancer Cell Replication

Normal breast tissue responds to changing hormone levels at puberty, during the menstrual cycle and during pregnancy. The ovarian steroid hormones oestrogen and progesterone are central to breast development and preparation for lactation, although these processes also involve hormones produced by the adrenal (glucocorticoids) and pituitary glands (growth hormone and prolactin) [11]. Some breast tumours remain responsive to these hormones, and hormone-responsive breast cancer cell lines provide well-characterised experimental models in which hormonal regulation of proliferation can be studied [1]. Although a distinguishing characteristic of these cells is their sensitivity to steroid hormones, responses to a broad spectrum of peptide hormones, growth factors and cytokines have also been recorded (Table 1). For some of these molecules, e.g. progestins [12], oestrogens [13] and 1,25 dihydroxyvitamin D_3 [14], both stimulation and inhibition have been observed, and the magnitude of the observed effect can vary widely, in part depending on the cell line and the culture conditions. Compounds which are stimulatory at low concentrations can be inhibitory at higher concentrations, e.g. oestrogen and 1,25 dihydroxyvitamin D_3. Progestins are able to both stimulate and inhibit proliferation within the same concentration range: although the dominant effect is growth inhibition, this is preceded by transient acceleration of progression through the cell cycle [12].

Although it does not represent an exhaustive survey, Table 1 illustrates one aspect of the complexity of the regulation of breast cancer cell growth, i.e., the number and diversity of molecules which can either stimulate or inhibit replication. This level of complexity identifies the immediate challenge of defining at the molecular level the inter-relationships between signal transduction pathways and the convergence of these pathways on the regulation of expression of key cell cycle regulatory genes. An additional level of complexity results from the interactions between different growth regulatory molecules. For example, responses to progestins and antioestrogens can be modulated by insulin or epidermal growth factor (EGF) [15,16]. Furthermore, many of the molecules listed in Table 1 are present in serum, a routine component of medium used to

Table 1. Responses of breast cancer cells to growth-regulatory molecules

Stimulation	Inhibition
Steroids/Retinoids	
Oestrogens	Oestrogens
Progestins (transient)	Progestins
Thyroid hormones	Retinoids
1,25 dihydroxyvitamin D_3	1,25 dihydroxyvitamin D_3
	Androgens
Growth factors	
Insulin-like growth factor-I, -II	Transforming growth factor β
Epidermal growth factor	Amphiregulin
Transforming growth factor α	Mammastatin
Acidic and basic fibroblast growth factor	Mammary-derived growth inhibitor
Mammary-derived growth factor	
Peptide hormones	
Insulin	Calcitonin
Prolactin	Somatostatin
Growth hormone	Melatonin
Cytokines	
Granulocyte-macrophage colony-stimulating factor	Interleukins 1, 4 & 6
	Interferons α, β & γ
	Tumour necrosis factor

culture breast cancer cell lines. This highlights the need to work under more defined conditions when attempting to better delineate the effects of individual growth regulatory molecules and define the molecular basis of their action [17,18].

To study the role of individual hormones or growth factors, we have employed chemically defined, serum-free medium to maintain breast cancer cell lines in a viable but non-proliferating state [17,18]. These cells can be stimulated to re-initiate cell cycle progression by the addition of a single agent. An example is shown in Figure 1 where T-47D cells which had been growth arrested in serum-free medium were treated with 10 µg/ml insulin to re-initiate cell cycle progression. Twelve hours after insulin stimulation, the proportion of cells in S phase (DNA synthesis) began to increase, reaching a plateau at 21-24 hours. Simultaneously the proportion of cells in G_1 began to decline (Fig. 1A). The stimulated cells subsequently completed DNA replication and divided. These data, obtained using analytical DNA flow cytometry, are complemented by studies monitoring the expression of known cell cycle regulated genes. Thus the induction of histone H4 gene expression, a marker of DNA synthesis, is identical with changes in % S-phase cells while the cell cycle phase-specific cyclin genes, cyclins A and B1, are induced in S phase and G_2, respectively (Fig. 1B). The significance of the induction of cyclin D1, a G_1 cyclin, is discussed later (see Mechanisms of Growth Control).

This system has allowed quantitative comparisons of various stimulatory agents by measuring the proportion of cells which enter S phase after treatment with different growth factors or hormones. Insulin, insulin-like growth factor-I (IGF-I) and basic fibroblast growth factor all stimulate a similar proportion of cells to enter S phase but both transforming growth factor α (TGFα) and EGF are less effective. All treatments lead to semi-synchronous entry into S phase after a lag period of about 10 hours [17,18]. The time-course of changes in cell cycle phase distribution for growth factor-stimulated cells is almost identical to that observed after mitotic selection of T-47D cells, indicating that these factors exert their effects on cell cycle progression early in G_1 phase (Fig. 2).

In serum-free medium, insulin is capable of eliciting a sustained response, leading to

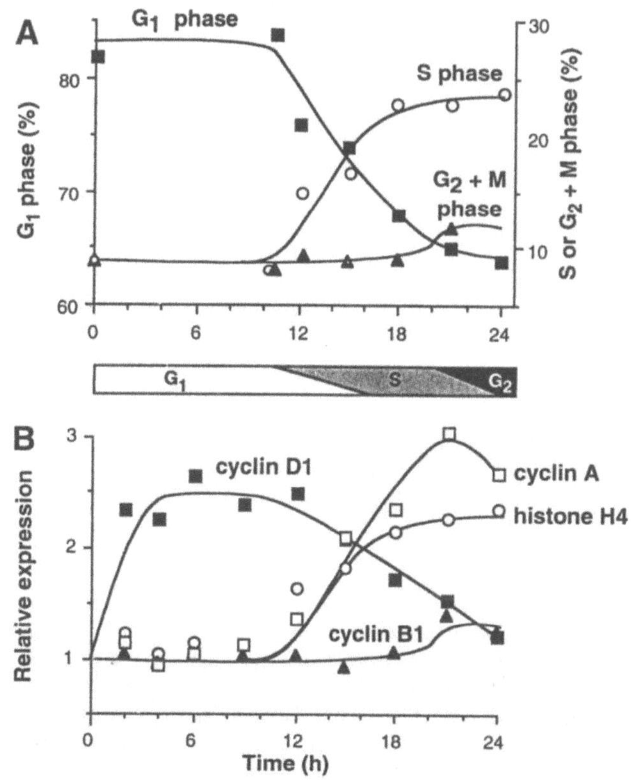

Fig. 1. Growth factor stimulation of cell cycle progression and cell cycle phase-specific gene expression in breast cancer cells. The hormone-responsive, human breast cancer cell line T-47D, growth arrested in chemically defined, serum-free medium, was stimulated to re-initiate cell cycle progression by addition of 10 µg/ml insulin at time 0. A. Temporal changes in cell cycle phase distribution as measured by analytical DNA flow cytometry depicting the proportion of G_1 (■), S (○) and G_2 + M (▲) phase cells. B. Temporal changes in mRNA levels for histone H4 (○) and cyclin D1 (■), A (□) and B1 (▲) genes.

growth rates only slightly slower than those achieved in the presence of serum [17,18]. This allows the actions of inhibitors of proliferation, for example antioestrogens and antiprogestins, to be studied in the presence of a single mitogen, insulin. Both steroids and steroid antagonists act within G_1 phase [12,19], where much of the control over progress through the mammalian cell division cycle is known to occur. Measuring the time at which changes in the proportion of cells entering S phase in treated cultures occur, allows some inferences to be drawn about the part of the cell cycle which is sensitive to individual compounds. These points of action can be more accurately identified in experiments utilising cells that have

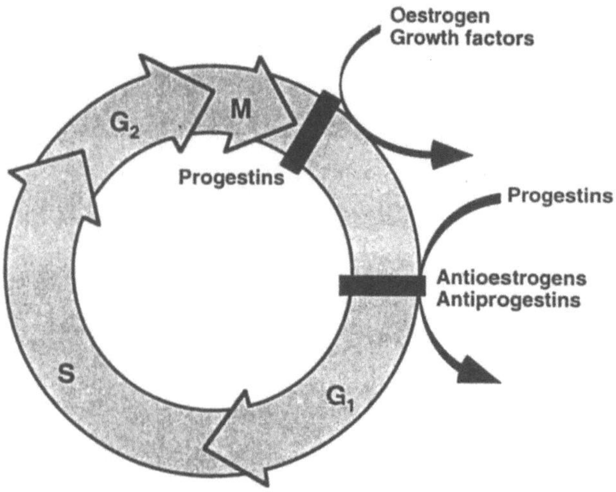

Fig. 2. A schematic representation of the cell division cycle and the approximate points of action of growth factors, steroids and steroid antagonists. The 4 phases of the cell cycle are illustrated, i.e. G_1, S or DNA synthesis, G_2 and mitosis. Growth factors including EGF, TGFα and bFGF exert their stimulatory effects early in G_1 phase. Oestrogen, in the absence of insulin or IGFs, is poorly mitogenic, appears to act at a similar point early in G_1 to stimulate cell cycle progression. In contrast, the stimulatory effect of progestin appears to occur later in G_1 at a point where antioestrogen and antiprogestin exert their inhibitory actions. The inhibitory effects of progestins are manifested very early in G_1.

been synchronised by mitotic selection [20, 21]. Figure 2 represents the approximate points of action within G_1 phase of the cell cycle, as identified by studies in this laboratory, for a series of growth factors, steroids and steroid antagonists. Sensitivity to the inhibitory effects of antioestrogens and antiprogestins occurs in approximately the same portion of G_1 [17]. As stated above, progestins have both stimulatory and inhibitory effects on breast cancer cell cycle progression and these phenomena have been studied in detail [12]. The stimulatory effect of progestins and the inhibitory effect of antiprogestins appear to result from opposing effects on a single pathway, while the inhibitory effect of progestins takes place much earlier in G_1 [12,17,22]. These studies identify multiple pathways used by different molecules to regulate breast cancer cell cycle progression.

Models for Steroid-Stimulated Growth

Breast cancer cells not only respond to many exogenous growth factors, but also synthesise and secrete growth factors, some of which are capable of autocrine stimulation of breast cancer proliferation or paracrine stimulation of neighbouring stromal cells. For example, TGFα is found in the conditioned medium of breast cancer cell lines at concentrations within the range required to stimulate their proliferation [1]. Furthermore, within tumours neighbouring stromal cells may produce growth factors which stimulate breast cancer cells. Although IGFs are amongst the most effective mitogens for these cells, mRNA specific for IGFs cannot be detected in the majority of hormone-responsive breast cancer cell lines, or in malignant breast epithelial cells [23]. However, stromal cells in tissue sections of breast cancer biopsies contain IGF-I mRNA [23]. Since the production of IGFs by stromal cells can be stimulated by TGFα and platelet-derived growth factor, which are produced and secreted by tumour cells, this may lead to the mutual dependence of epithelial and stromal cells within the tumour. Such a mechanism may be implicated in the acquisition of autonomous growth and the development of endocrine resistance [24].

Because production of some growth factors, either by breast cancer cells or by stromal cells, is regulated by oestrogen, it has been proposed that these growth factors mediate the effects of oestrogen on proliferation [1]. Although this suggestion, the "autocrine hypothesis", has been widely supported to the point that it is accepted as dogma in many recent publications, the data supporting such conclusions are not strong and indeed there is convincing evidence against such a model [25]. For example, although TGFα or IGF-I induction of proliferation was prevented by antibodies which blocked binding of the growth factor to its receptor, the same antibodies had little effect on oestrogen induction of proliferation [26]. Furthermore, mitogenic peptide growth factors elicit a cascade of responses which transmit signals from their receptors to the cell nucleus. One step in this cascade is thought to be activation of ribosomal S6 kinase. However, although peptide growth factors lead to the activation of this kinase in breast cancer cells, it is not activated in response to mitogenic concentrations of oestrogen [27]. These and other data argue that the well-studied growth factors EGF, TGFα and IGF-I do not mediate mitogenic responses to oestrogen. However, it is likely that these growth factors act together with oestrogen in the overall control of breast cancer cell proliferation. Indeed, they appear to synergise with oestrogen to stimulate proliferation [28,29]. Similar arguments for a role of autocrine peptides in the control of progestin-induced cell proliferation have also been proposed [30]. Again there is strong evidence that progestins regulate the levels of expression of EGF, TGFα, TGFß and the EGF receptor in human breast cancer cells [12,30,31] but it is likely that this is a consequence rather than the cause of changes in the rate of cell cycle progression. Data from this laboratory [12] provide convincing evidence that progestin stimulation of cell cycle progression results in cells entering S phase several hours before cells stimulated with EGF or TGFα, precluding the possibility that progestin-induced increases in expression or activation of these growth factors is an essential component of the proliferative response to progestins (Fig. 3A).

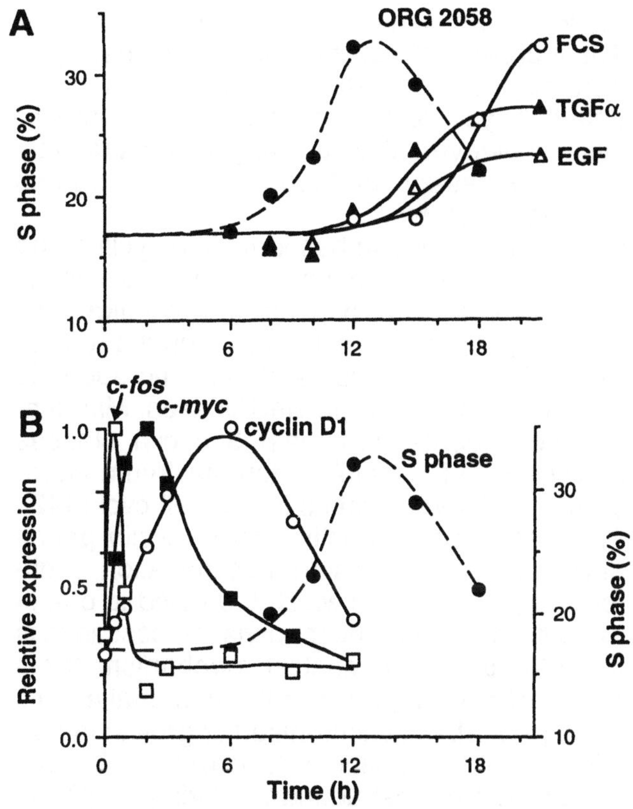

Fig. 3. Progestin and growth factor stimulation of cell cycle progression and expression of cell cycle regulatory genes in breast cancer cells. A. T-47D cells growing in serum-free medium supplemented with insulin were further stimulated with progestin (●), EGF (Δ), TGFα (▲) or foetal calf serum (FCS, ○), and the increase in the rate of cell cycle progression monitored by measuring % S phase cells. B. Progestin treatment resulted in an increase in the rate of cell cycle traverse which was accompanied by induction of the cell cycle regulatory genes *c-fos* (□), *c-myc* (■) and cyclin D1 (○) which preceded progression into S phase (●).

Mechanisms of Growth Control

Within the last decade substantial advances have been made in understanding molecular mechanisms which underlie progress through the cell cycle. It is likely that a small number of "cell division cycle" genes control transition from one stage of the cell cycle to the next and that these genes or their products are activated by mitogens including both growth factors and steroid hormones. Some candidate genes have been identified, but it is not clear whether all cells share the same regulatory mechanisms: indeed there is accumulating evidence for cell-specific utilisation of some of these genes [32,33]. The basic biological data now available can be used to begin identifying key cell cycle regulatory genes for normal and neoplastic epithelial cells. One approach is to study genes for which there is evidence of regulatory roles in other systems. For example, it is now well documented that the initiation of proliferation is accompanied by the induction of a large number of immediate-early genes which are characterised by rapid induction without a requirement for protein synthesis. These include the nuclear proto-oncogenes *c-fos* and *c-myc*, necessary for progress through G_1 phase [34,35]. In breast cancer cells, stimulation by oestrogen or progestin (Fig. 3) is accompanied by rapid but transient increases in *c-fos* and *c-myc* expression [12,36-38]. Simultaneous treatment with a progestin and an antiprogestin prevents both the stimulation of entry into S-phase and the stimulation of *c-myc* expression [12]. Both antioestrogen and antiprogestin inhibition of insulin-induced cell cycle progression in T-47D cells is accompanied by a rapid depletion of *c-myc* mRNA [38,39]. In addition, if the induction of *c-myc* by oestrogen is prevented by antisense oligonucleotides, no relative increase in cell number after oestrogen treatment is seen [40]. Thus, c-*myc* is a candidate cell cycle regulatory gene in breast cancer cells. However, it is unlikely to be the only gene necessary for these cells to progress through G_1 phase.

Recent investigation has identified cyclins and cyclin-dependent kinases (cdks) as key regulators of cell cycle progression in eukaryotic cells [41,42]. These molecules form the regulatory subunits (cyclins) and catalytic subunits (cdks) of cell cycle-regulated kinases. Mammalian cells contain at least 5 cyclin classes (cyclins A to E), which reach maximum abundance at different points in the cell cycle [42]. The transcriptional activation of cyclin genes and consequent transient accumulation of different cyclin proteins which then bind to one of the cdks to initiate phosphorylation cascades is thought to be the central mechanism for a series of control points in the mammalian cell cycle [41,42]. In synchronised or growth factor-stimulated mammalian cells, cyclins C, D1, D2, D3 and E are most abundant during G_1 phase [32,43,44], suggesting that these cyclins may function at G_1 control points in mammalian cells. Similarly, sequential induction of cyclins D1 (early G_1 phase), D3, E, A (late G_1/early S phase) and B1 (G_2 phase) was observed following insulin stimulation of T-47D cell cycle progression in serum-free medium (Fig. 1B) [39]. A similar pattern of cyclin gene expression was observed in EGF-stimulated normal breast epithelial cells [45]. These latter data identify G_1 cyclins as potential targets for hormonal regulation of breast epithelial cell proliferation.

Evidence that cyclin D1 is an early response to mitogenic stimulation of T-47D breast cancer cells (Fig. 1B) suggests a function at a time compatible with the actions of steroids and steroid antagonists (Fig. 2). Transient acceleration of G_1 phase cells by progestin was also accompanied by rapid induction of cyclin D1 within 2 hours (Fig. 3B). The time-course of induction of cyclin D1 and the ability of delayed administration of the antiprogestin RU 486 to antagonise progestin-induced increases in both cyclin D1 mRNA and entry into S phase support a central role for cyclin D1 in mediating progestin stimulation in T-47D cells [39]. These data demonstrate that changes in cyclin D1 gene expression are often associated with changes in the rate of T-47D breast cancer cell cycle progression and suggest that this gene may have a key regulatory role in breast cell cycle control.

Potential Mechanisms for Loss of Normal Growth Control

The data summarised above define a number of growth regulatory molecules which mediate their effects on cell cycle progression via their respective receptors and signal transduction pathways, ultimately influencing the level of expression of key regulatory genes, potentially including c-*myc* and cyclin D1, to control rates of breast epithelial cell cycle progression. Thus the loss of normal regulation of the expression or function of genes involved in any of these steps might be expected to lead to the loss of normal growth control and confer some growth advantage perhaps by acquisition of autonomous growth control or loss of normal steroidal control of cell cycle progression. Reference to known genetic abnormalities present in human breast tumours supports this hypothesis. Table 2 summarises a series of genes which are commonly amplified, overexpressed, deleted or mutated in human breast cancer. It is of considerable interest and likely functional significance that the majority of these genes encode either receptor tyrosine kinases, which mediate the effects of growth regulatory peptides involved in the normal control of breast epithelial cell proliferation, or nuclear proto-oncogenes and tumour suppressor genes known to be intimately involved in cell cycle control. Since the role of many of these genes in the development and progression of breast cancer has been reviewed recently [46-49], the remainder of this review will focus on c-*myc* and cyclin D1 which appear to be intimately involved in steroidal control of cell proliferation.

Support for a role for c-*myc* activation in the development of breast cancer comes from evidence for common amplification and/or overexpression of c-*myc* in breast tumours [50, and refs. therein]. Amplification of c-*myc* is generally found in about 20% of breast carcinomas, with an association sometimes found with steroid hormone receptor status, i.e., amplification is usually associated with the absence of steroid

Table 2. Potential oncogenes and tumour suppressor genes that are commonly amplified, overexpressed, deleted or mutated in human breast cancer

Growth factors	
int-2/FGF3	amplified but not expressed
hst-1/FGF4	amplified but not expressed
Growth factor receptors	
c-*erb*B-1/EGF-R	overexpressed
c-*erb*B-2/HER-2/*neu*	amplified and/or overexpressed
c-*flg*/FGFR1	amplified
c-*bek*/FGFR2	amplified
Cell cycle regulatory genes	
c-*myc*, c-*myb*	amplified and/or overexpressed
cyclin D1/*PRAD*1	amplified and/or overexpressed
RB, p53	deleted and mutated

receptors [50] and poor prognosis [51]. Whether the poor prognosis associated with c-*myc* amplification reflects resistance to endocrine therapy is unclear. In experimental models of mammary tumourigenesis, some studies have shown that increased expression of *myc* is related to increased tumourigenesis [52,53], while others have concluded that *myc* overexpression is insufficient for malignant transformation [54]. Transgenic mice expressing c-*myc* under the control of hormonally-inducible promoters develop mammary adenocarcinomas in conjunction with pregnancy [55]. In sublines of a human breast cancer cell line, SW 613-S, which have variable levels of c-*myc* amplification, high levels of amplification are associated with tumourigenicity in nude mice [52]. The ER-negative cell lines BT 20 and MDA-MB-231 constitutively express high levels of c-*myc* mRNA, in the absence of amplification of the gene, also suggesting that overexpression of c-*myc* may be associated with the more highly tumourigenic, hormone-independent phenotype [36]. However, constitutive overexpression of transfected c-*myc* sequences does not confer E_2-independence on MCF-7 cells injected into nude mice [56]: in fact, overexpression of c-*myc* was inhibitory rather than stimulatory of growth. However, interpretation of this result may be complicated by evidence for poor cell survival after induction of high levels of c-*myc* protein [57] due perhaps to the role of Myc in inducing apoptotic cell death [58]. Interestingly, oestrogen withdrawal of MCF-7 tumours in nude mice results in c-*myc* induction and apoptosis [59] and treatment with antioestrogen or antiprogestin has been reported to have apoptotic effects on the same cells in culture [60].

There is, as yet, no direct evidence for transforming potential of the mammalian cyclin genes. However, as likely mediators of mitogen/growth inhibitor action in G_1 phase, the G_1 cyclins (C, D1-3 and E) and associated kinase partners have a potential role in carcinogenesis and tumour progression and in the development of hormone resistance. Overexpression of these genes might be expected to result in increased proliferative drive whereas this is less likely for the mitotic cyclins whose destruction is required for further cell cycle progression to occur [42].

Cyclin D1 is a strong candidate oncogene [44] and is the protein product of the *BCL*1 (= *PRAD*1) locus, which maps to chromosome 11q13 [44, 61]. This region is amplified in 15-20% of breast cancers [62,63]. Unlike the FGF3 and FGF4 genes, which are also within the 11q13 amplicon, cyclin D1 and the recently identified EMS1 gene are commonly expressed in breast tumours [64-66]. Overexpression is due to mechanisms other than amplification in some tumours [65] and cell lines [66]. We have recently studied cyclin mRNA expression in an extensive series of breast cancer cell lines and tumour biopsies. Fifty-six of 124 tumours (45%) expressed cyclin D1 mRNA at levels above the maximum observed in histologically normal breast tissue [66]. Those tumours forming the group with the highest expression of cyclin D1 were uniformly EGF receptor-negative and ER-positive, expressing significantly higher ER levels than tumours with lower cyclin D1 levels. This observation is in accord with previous studies that show an association between cyclin D1 amplification and ER-positivity [67]. Thus 11q13 amplification and perhaps cyclin D1 overexpression identify a subgroup of ER-positive tumours with lymph node involvement [62] and a poor prognosis [68]. It remains to be determined whether the latter association [68] is the result of greater tumour aggressiveness or resistance to adjuvant therapy.

Among breast cancer cell lines, cyclin D1 amplification or high expression is not related to ER positivity, in contrast to tumours. Of 20 cell lines, high expression of cyclin D1 was detected in 5 lines and gene amplification in 6 [66]. Overexpression occurred in both the presence and absence of gene amplification and conversely, amplification did not invariably lead to overexpression. It is not clear whether any of the ER-positive cell lines with cyclin D1 overexpression represents a model for ER-positive but poor prognosis tumours. The common amplification and concurrent overexpression of cyclin D1 in tumours and cell lines suggests this may be an important gene contributing to tumour development and/or progression. However, it has yet to be determined whether cyclin D1 gene dysregulation is an early or late event in the evolution of the malignant phenotype and what the relationship is between expression and the steroid hormone responsive phenotype. Our results showing rapid down-regulation of cyclin D1 mRNA by antioestrogen in breast cancer cells [39] suggest that overexpression of this cyclin is a potential mechanism for antioestrogen resistance.

Summary and Conclusions

Analysis of factors that control breast cancer cell proliferation has identified the involvement of a broad spectrum of hormones, growth factors and cytokines. Data on the cell cycle phase-specific action of some of these regulatory molecules have facilitated the development of hypotheses as to which cell cycle regulatory genes may be the downstream targets for proliferative control in breast epithelium. To date the nuclear proto-oncogene, c-*myc,* and the cell cycle regulatory G_1 cyclin, cyclin D1, have been identified as potential candidates. The corollary to this hypothesis is that dysregulated function of these genes or indeed the function of any genes involved in transmitting signals from receptors to the nucleus to regulate the expression of these key regulatory genes may lead to aberrant growth control. This in turn may contribute to tumourigenesis and/or tumour progression including the loss of steroid responsiveness and the development of antioestrogen resistance. The known mitogenic role of EGF, TGFα and bFGF and the common overexpression of their receptors in breast tumour biopsies support this view [49,69]. Further developments in our understanding of receptors, signal transduction pathways and cell cycle control in normal and neoplastic breast epithelium is likely to have direct impact on clinical breast cancer through the identification of new prognostic markers and the development of novel therapeutic strategies targeted to these pathways.

Acknowledgments

Research in this laboratory is supported by grants from the National Health and Medical Research Council of Australia; the New South Wales State Cancer Council, the Leo and Jenny Leukaemia and Cancer Foundation and MLC Life Ltd.

REFERENCES

1 Dickson RB and Lippman ME: Estrogenic regulation of growth and polypeptide growth factor secretion in human breast carcinoma. Endocr Rev 1987 (8):29-43

2 Van de Vijver MJ and Nusse R: The molecular biology of breast cancer. Biochim Biophys Acta 1991 (1072):33-50

3 Henderson B, Ross R and Bernstein L: Estrogens as a cause of human cancer: the Richard and Hinda Rosenthal Foundation Award lecture. Cancer Res 1988 (48):246-253

4 Clarke GM and McGuire WL: Steroid receptors and other prognostic factors in primary breast cancer. Semin Oncol 1988 (15):20-25

5 Nayfield SG, Karp JE, Ford LG, Dorr FA and Kramer BS: Potential role of tamoxifen in prevention of breast cancer. JNCI 1991 (83):1450-1459

6 Early Breast Cancer Trialists' Collaborative Group: Systemic treatment of early breast cancer by hormonal, cytotoxic, or immune therapy. Lancet 1992 (339):1-15, 71-85

7 Katzenellenbogen BK: Antiestrogen resistance: Mechanisms by which breast cancer cells undermine the effectiveness of endocrine therapy. JNCI 1991 (83):1434-1435

8 Horwitz KB: The molecular biology of RU 486. Is there a role for antiprogestins in the treatment of breast cancer? Endocr Rev 1992 (13):146-163

9 Smith MA, Parkinson DR, Cheson BD and Friedman MA: Retinoids in cancer therapy. J Clin Oncol 1992 (10):839-864

10 Pastan I and FitzGerald D: Recombinant toxins for cancer treatment. Science 1991 (254):1173-1177

11 Russo J and Russo IH: Development of the human mammary gland. In: Neville MC and Daniels CW (eds) The Mammary Gland. Development, Regulation and Function. Plenum Press, New York 1987 pp 67-93

12 Musgrove EA, Lee CSL and Sutherland RL: Progestins both stimulate and inhibit breast cancer cell cycle progression while increasing expression of transforming growth factor α, epidermal growth factor receptor, *c-fos* and *c-myc* genes. Mol Cell Biol 1991 (11):5032-5043

13 Reddel RR and Sutherland RL: Effects of pharmacological concentrations of estrogens on proliferation and cell cycle kinetics of human breast cancer cell lines in vitro. Cancer Res 1987 (47):5323-5329

14 Eisman JA, Sutherland RL, McMenemy ML, Fragonas JC, Musgrove EA and Pang GY: Effects of 1,25-dihydroxyvitamin D3 on cell-cycle kinetics of T 47D human breast cancer cells. J Cell Physiol 1989 (138):611-616

15 Sarup JC, Rao KV and Fox CF: Decreased progesterone binding and attenuated progesterone action in cultured human breast carcinoma cells treated with epidermal growth factor. Cancer Res 1988 (48):5071-5078

16 Koga M, Musgrove EA and Sutherland RL: Modulation of the growth-inhibitory effects of progestins and the antiestrogen hydroxyclomiphene on human breast cancer cells by epidermal growth factor and insulin. Cancer Res 1989 (49):112-116

17 Sutherland RL, Lee CSL, Feldman RS and Musgrove EA: Regulation of breast cancer cell cycle progression by growth factors, steroids and steroid antagonists. J Steroid Biochem Molec Biol 1992 (41):315-321

18 Musgrove EA and Sutherland RL: Acute effects of growth factors on T-47D breast cancer cell cycle progression. Submitted

19 Musgrove EA and Sutherland RL: Steroids, growth factors and cell cycle controls in breast cancer. In: Lippman ME and Dickson RB (eds) Regulatory Mechanisms in Breast Cancer. Kluwer Academic Publishers, Boston 1991 pp 305-331

20 Taylor IW, Hodson PJ, Green MD and Sutherland RL: Effects of tamoxifen on cell cycle progression of synchronous MCF-7 human mammary carcinoma cells. Cancer Res 1983 (43):4007-4010

21 Musgrove EA, Wakeling AE and Sutherland RL: Points of action of estrogen antagonists and a calmodulin antagonist within the MCF-7 human breast cancer cell cycle. Cancer Res 1989 (49):2398-2404

22 Sutherland RL, Hall RE, Pang GYN, Musgrove EA and Clarke CL: Effect of medroxyprogesterone acetate on proliferation and cell cycle kinetics of human mammary carcinoma cells. Cancer Res 1988 (48):5084-5091

23 Yee D, Rosen N, Favoni RE and Cullen KJ: The insulin-like growth factors, their receptors, and their binding proteins in human breast cancer. In: Lippman ME and Dickson RB (eds) Regulatory Mechanisms in Breast Cancer. Kluwer Academic Publishers, Boston 1991 pp 93-106

24 Daly RJ, deFazio A, Watts CKW, Musgrove EA and Sutherland RL: Steroids, steroid antagonists and cell cycle progression. In: Dickson RB and Lippman ME (eds) Drug and Hormonal Resistance in Breast Cancer: Cellular and Molecular Mechanisms. Ellis Horwood, Chichester 1993 (in press)

25 van der Burg B, de Groot RP, Isbrucker L, Kruijer W and de Laat SW: Direct stimulation by estrogen of growth factor signal transduction pathways in human breast cancer cells. J Steroid Biochem Molec Biol 1992 (43):111-115

26 Arteaga CL and Osborne CK: Growth factors as mediators of estrogen/antioestrogen action in human breast cancer cells. In: Lippman ME and Dickson RB (eds) Regulatory Mechanisms in Breast Cancer. Kluwer Academic Publishers, Boston 1991 pp 289-304

27 Novak-Hofer I, Küng W, Fabbro D and Eppenberger U: Estrogen stimulates growth of mammary tumor cells ZR-75 without activation of S6 kinase and S6 phosphorylation. Difference from epidermal growth factor and α-transforming growth-factor-induced proliferation. Eur J Biochem 1987 (164):445-451

28 van der Burg B, Rutteman GR, Blankenstein MA, de Laat SW and van Zoelen EJJ: Mitogenic stimulation of human breast cancer cells in a growth factor-defined medium: synergistic action of insulin and estrogen. J Cell Physiol 1988 (134):101-108

29 Stewart AJ, Westley BR and May FEB: Modulation of the proliferative response of breast cancer cells

to growth factors by estrogen. Br J Cancer 1992 (66):640-648
30 Murphy LC, Dotzlaw H, Alkalaf M, Coutts A, Miller T, Wong MSJ, Gong Y and Murphy LJ: Mechanisms of growth inhibition by antiestrogens and progestins in human breast cancer cells. J Steroid Biochem Molec Biol 1992 (43):117-121
31 Murphy LC and Dotzlaw H: Regulation of transforming growth factor α and transforming growth factor ß messenger ribonucleic acid abundance in T-47D, human breast cancer cells. Mol Endocrinol 1989 (3):611-617
32 Matsushime H, Roussel MF, Ashmun RA and Sherr CJ: Colony-stimulating factor 1 regulates novel cyclins during the G1 phase of the cell cycle. Cell 1991 (65):701-713
33 Inaba T, Matsushime H, Valentine M, Roussel MF, Sherr CJ and Look AT: Genomic organization, chromosomal localization, and independent expression of human cyclin D genes. Genomics 1992 (13):565-574
34 Holt JT, Venkat Gopal T, Moulton AD and Nienhuis AW: Inducible production of *c-fos* antisense RNA inhibits 3T3 cell proliferation. Proc Natl Acad Sci 1986 (83):4794-4798
35 Heikkila R, Schwab G, Wickstrom E, Loke SL, Pluznik DH, Watt R and Neckers LM: A *c-myc* antisense oligodeoxynucleotide inhibits entry into S phase but not progress from G_0 to G_1. Nature 1987 (328):445-449
36 Dubik D, Dembinski TC and Shiu RPC: Stimulation of *c-myc* oncogene expression associated with estrogen-induced proliferation of human breast cancer cells. Cancer Res 1987 (47):6517-6521
37 Wilding G, Lippman ME and Gelmann EP: Effects of steroid hormones and peptide growth factors on protooncogene *c-fos* expression in human breast cancer cells. Cancer Res 1988 (48):802-805
38 Wong MSJ and Murphy LC: Differential regulation of *c-myc* by progestins and antiestrogens in T-47D human breast cancer cells. J Steroid Biochem Molec Biol 1991 (39):39-44
39 Musgrove EA, Hamilton JA, Lee CSL, Sweeney KJE, Watts CKW and Sutherland RL: Growth factor, steroid and steroid antagonist regulation of cyclin gene expression associated with changes in T-47D human breast cancer cell cycle progression. Mol Cell Biol 1993 (in press)
40 Watson PH, Pon RT and Shiu RPC: Inhibition of *c-myc* expression by phosphorothioate antisense oligonucleotide identifies a critical role for *c-myc* in the growth of human breast cancer. Cancer Res 1991 (51):3996-4000
41 Nurse P: Universal control mechanism regulating onset of M-phase. Nature 1990 (344):503-508
42 Hunter T and Pines J: Cyclins and cancer. Cell 1991 (66):1071-1074
43 Lew DJ, Dulic V and Reed SI: Isolation of three novel human cyclins by rescue of G1 cyclin (Cln) function in yeast. Cell 1991 (66):1197-1206
44 Motokura T, Bloom T, Kim HG, Jüppner H, Ruderman J, Kronenberg H and Arnold A: A novel cyclin encoded by a *bcl1*-linked candidate oncogene. Nature 1991 (350):512-515
45 Motokura T, Keyomarsi K, Kronenberg HM and Arnold A: Cloning and characterization of human cyclin D3, a cDNA closely related in sequence to the PRAD1/cyclin D1 proto-oncogene. J Biol Chem 1992 (267):20412-20415
46 Gullick WJ: The role of the epidermal growth factor receptor and the c-erbB-2 protein in breast cancer. Int J Cancer 1990 (Suppl. 5):55-61
47 Lee EY-HP, Bookstein R and Lee W-H: Role of the retinoblastoma gene in the oncogenesis of human breast carcinoma. In: Lippman ME and Dickson RB (eds) Regulatory Mechanisms in Breast Cancer. Kluwer Academic Publishers, Boston 1991 pp 23-43
48 Harris AL: p53 expression in human breast cancer. Adv Cancer Res 1992 (59):69-88
49 Klijn JGM, Berns EMJJ, Schmitz PIM and Foekens JA: The clinical significance of epidermal growth factor receptor (EGF-R) in human breast cancer: a review on 5232 patients. Endocr Rev 1992 (13):3-17
50 Berns EMJJ, Klijn JGN, van Staveren IL, Portengen H, Noordegraaf E and Foekens JA: Prevalence of amplification of the oncogenes *c-myc*, *HER2/neu*, and *int-2* in one thousand human breast tumours: correlation with steroid receptors. Eur J Cancer 1992 (28):697-700
51 Berns EMJJ, Klijn JGM, van Putten WLJ, van Staveren IL, Portengen H and Foekens JA: *c-myc* amplification is a better prognostic factor than *HER2/neu* amplification in primary breast cancer. Cancer Res 1992 (52):1107-1113
52 Lavialle C, Modjtahedi N, Lamonerie T, Frebourg T, Landin R-M, Fossar N, Lhomond G, Cassingena R and Brison O: The human breast carcinoma cell line SW 613-S: an experimental system to study tumor heterogeneity in relation to *c-myc* amplification, growth factor production and other markers. Anticancer Res 1989 (9):1265-1279
53 Telang NT, Osborne MP, Sweterlitsch LA and Narayanan R: Neoplastic transformation of mouse mammary epithelial cells by deregulated *myc* expression. Cell Regulation 1990 (1):863-872
54 Edwards PAW, Ward JL and Bradbury JM: Alteration of morphogenesis by the *v-myc* oncogene in transplants of mammary gland. Oncogene 1988 (2):407-412
55 Stewart TA, Pattengale PK and Leder P: Spontaneous mammary adenocarcinomas in transgenic mice that carry and express MTV/*myc* fusion genes. Cell 1984 (38):627-637
56 Liu E, Santos G, Lee WM, Osborne CK and Benz CC: Effects of *c-myc* overexpression on the growth characteristics of MCF-7 human breast cancer cells. Oncogene 1989 (4):979-984
57 Wurm FM, Gwinn KA and Kingston RE: Inducible overproduction of the mouse *c-myc* protein in mammalian cells. Proc Natl Acad Sci 1986 (83):5414-5418
58 Evan GI, Wyllie AH, Gilbert CS, Littlewood TD, Land H, Brooks M, Waters CM, Penn LZ and Hancock DC: Induction of apoptosis in fibroblasts by *c-myc* protein. Cell 1992 (69):119-128
59 Kyprianou N, English HF, Davidson NE and Isaacs JT: Programmed cell death during regression of the MCF-7 human breast cancer following estrogen ablation. Cancer Res 1991 (51):162-166

60 Bardon S, Vignon F, Montcourrier P and Rochefort H: Steroid receptor-mediated cytotoxicity of an antiestrogen and an antiprogestin in breast cancer cells. Cancer Res 1987 (47):1441-1448

61 Withers DA, Harvey RC, Faust JB, Melnyk O, Carey K and Meeker TC: Characterization of a candidate *bcl-1* gene. Mol Cell Biol 1991 (11):4846-4853

62 Adnane J, Gaudray P, Simon M-P, Simony-Lafontaine J, Jeanteur P and Theillet C: Proto-oncogene amplification and human breast tumor phenotype. Oncogene 1989 (4):1389-1395

63 Ali IU, Merlo G, Callahan R and Lidereau R: The amplification unit on chromosome 11q13 in aggressive primary human breast tumors entails the *bcl*-1, *int*-2 and *hst* loci. Oncogene 1989 (4):89-92

64 Lammie GA, Fantl V, Smith R, Schuuring E, Brookes S, Michalides R, Dickson C, Arnold A and Peters G: D11S287, a putative oncogene on chromosome 11q13, is amplified and expressed in squamous cell and mammary carcinomas and linked to BCL-1. Oncogene 1991 (6):439-444

65 Schuuring E, Verhoeven E, Mooi WJ and Michalides RJAM: Identification and cloning of two overexpressed genes, U21B31/*PRAD1* and *EMS1*, within the amplified chromosome 11q13 region in human carcinomas. Oncogene 1992 (7):355-366

66 Buckley MF, Sweeney KJE, Hamilton JA, Sini RL, Manning DL, Nicholson RI, deFazio A, Watts CKW, Musgrove EA and Sutherland RL: Expression and amplification of cyclin genes in human breast cancer. Oncogene 1993 (in press)

67 Fantl V, Richards MA, Smith R, Lammie GA, Johnstone G, Allen D, Gregory W, Peters G, Dickson C and Barnes DM: Gene amplification on chromosome band 11q13 and oestrogen receptor status in breast cancer. Eur J Cancer 1990 (26):423-429

68 Schuuring E, Verhoeven E, van Tinteren H, Peterse JL, Nunnink B, Thunnissen FBJM, Devilee P, Cornelisse CJ, van de Vijver MJ, Mooi WJ and Michalides RJAM: Amplification of genes within the chromosome 11q13 region is indicative of poor prognosis in patients with operable breast cancer. Cancer Res 1992 (52):5229-5234

69 Adnane J, Gaudray P, Dionne CA, Crumley G, Jaye M, Schlessinger J, Jeanteur P, Birnbaum D and Theillet C: BEK and FLG, two receptors to members of the FGF family, are amplified in subsets of human breast cancers. Oncogene 1991 (6):659-663

Cyclical Activity and 'Ageing' of the Human Breast: Clues to Assessment of Risk and Strategies for Prevention

Anthony Howell [1], Elizabeth Anderson [2], Ian Laidlaw [1], Ana Schor [1], Seth Schor [3] and Christopher Potten [4]

1 CRC Department of Medical Oncology, Christie Hospital
2 Tumour Biochemistry Laboratory, Christie Hospital, Wilmslow Road, Manchester M20 9BX
4 Department of Epithelial Cell Biology, Paterson Institute for Cancer Research, Wilmslow Road, Manchester M20 9BX
3 Department of Cell and Structural Biology, University of Manchester, Manchester, United Kingdom

There is strong epidemiological evidence that environmental, hormonal and genetic factors affect the risk and development of breast cancer [1,2]. Migrant studies demonstrate that diet and culture are, in some way, related to the high incidence of breast cancer in 'westernised' societies. In addition, dietary and cultural factors may interact with hormonal risk factors since nutrition affects the age of menarche and social mores affect age of first birth [3]. However, in Western Europe and the United States most women live in similar environments and have diets which do not appear to be sufficiently different to alter risk appreciably [4,5]. Also the important endocrine risk factors often cancel each other out in individuals so that increased risk associated with an early menarche may be offset by the decreased risk associated with early childbirth. Discovery of genes associated with hereditary breast cancer are important advances but this type of breast cancer accounts for less than 5% of the total [6]. Thus the known risk factors appear to account for the variation in the incidence of breast cancer between but not within populations. The question arises: if within a population women have largely similar risk factors, why does breast cancer develop in some and not in others? Unless there are - as yet undiscovered - potent risk factors, it seems reasonable to suggest that there may be wide differences in the susceptibility of the breast to the putative environmental and hormonal influences which cause the disease.

The major functional unit of the breast is the lobule, which arises from a terminal duct and is comprised of several small blind-ending ductules (acini) lined by 2 layers of epithelial cells (luminal and myoepithelial). The terminal duct and ductules are surrounded by a specialised mesenchyme (intralobular stroma) and the epithelial structures and mesenchyme together form the terminal duct lobular units (TDLU). Careful histological studies indicate that most breast cancers arise from luminal epithelial cells within the TDLU (for discussion see [7]). The epithelial structures are not only intimately associated with their related mesenchyme but there is strong evidence which indicates that epithelial function depends upon reciprocal interactions between the two [8,9]. Variation in the susceptibility of the breast to environmental factors and endogenous influences between individuals may therefore be related to differences in the responsiveness of the epithelium, the mesenchyme or in their reciprocal interactions.

Although the known risk factors for breast cancer do not allow us to predict risk accurately, they do give clues concerning factors which might predispose luminal epithelial cells in the TDLU to neoplastic transformation. For example, the breast is more susceptible to radiation-induced cancer in females before age 20 (data summarised in [1]) and prolonged cyclical activity of the breast without interruption by pregnancy increases susceptibility (data summarised in [10,2]). These observations give rise to the question why the young breast is more susceptible and why cyclical activity of the breast predisposes to malignancy. The susceptibility of the young breast suggests

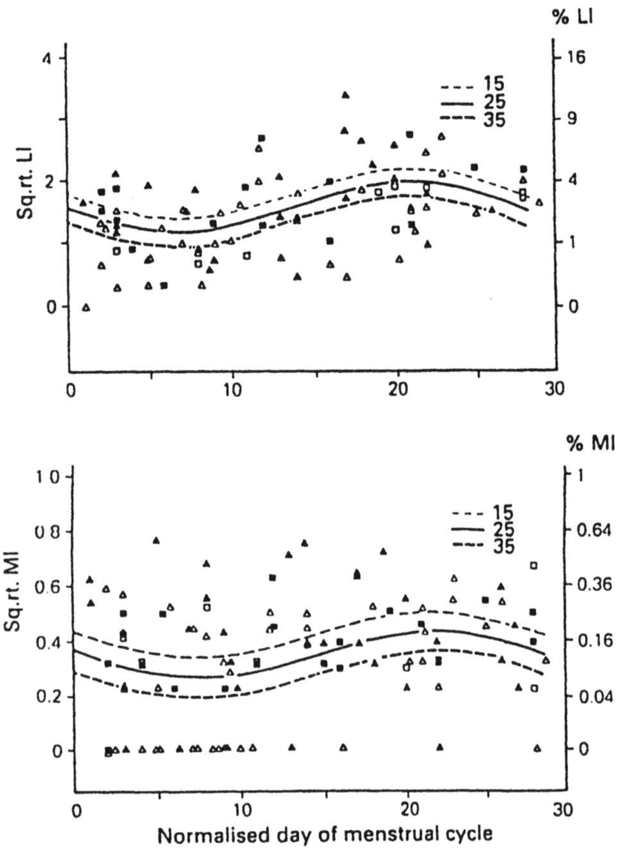

Fig. 1. The relationship between the day of the menstrual cycle and the thymidine labelling index (LI) and mitotic index (MI) in luminal epithelial cells of TDLUs. ▲ <25 years off the pill, ■ <25 years on the pill, Δ ≥25 years off the pill, □ ≥25 years on the pill. Because the LI also changed with age the values were normalised to age 15, 25 and 35 years and the predicted best fit curves shown for each age.

that risk is reduced with age and has led to the concept of breast ageing introduced by Pike et al. [11]. The importance of the menstrual cycle has led to several investigations on the human breast attempting to discern possible important changes in its structure and function during the cycle which could predispose to malignant change.

Here we will review data concerning the reported changes in the epithelium and mesenchyme of the TDLU with age and during the menstrual cycle which might be related to the subsequent risk of breast cancer. These considerations are not solely of academic interest since knowledge of the reasons for the differences in susceptibility between breasts may lead to more precise markers of risk and new approaches to breast cancer prevention: prediction of risk has increased in importance with the advent of chemoprevention trials. Also, these data may give insights concerning how we can detect the effects of chemopreventive agents on the breast which may provide important surrogate endpoints in these trials.

Changes in the Epithelium During the Menstrual Cycle

Several studies indicate that the rate of proliferation of the luminal epithelial cells of the TDLU is at its nadir during the mid-follicular phase and at its peak during the mid-luteal phase of the menstrual cycle, whether proliferation was measured by 3H thymidine labelling index (LI) or by mitotic index (MI) [12-17] (Fig. 1). These data were obtained from examination of histologically normal TDLU removed during reduction mammoplasties and at operation for removal of fibroadenomas. At each time point there is marked variation in LI and MI. For example, some of the highest LIs were seen in the mid-luteal phase of the cycle but even at this time some breasts showed little proliferation as exemplified by LIs of less than 1% in some samples: it is possible that differences in proliferation may relate to differences in risk. We estimated that age and day of cycle contributed only 10 to 25% to the variation seen in the data. Some variation is due to technical errors but differences in lobule sensitivity to circulating hormones may account for the remainder.

Morphological differences in the luminal and myoepithelial cells of the TDLU in the follicular and luteal phases of the cycle have been reported by several groups [15,18,19]. In the early follicular phase, the epithelium of the lobule appears to consist of a single cell layer with occasional basal cells. As the cycle continues into the luteal phase, the 2-layered structure of the epithelium becomes more evident; the luminal cells swell and show evidence of secretory activity; increased rough endoplasmic reticulum, a prominent Golgi complex and surface microvilli and budding. The basal myoepithelial cells develop an abundant clear vacuolated cytoplasm. In the early part of the cycle the lumen of the lobules is inconspicuous but gradually opens up and contains secretory material by the luteal phase. Material

with the electron microscopic appearance of glycogen appears in the luminal cells and in the vacuoles of the myoepithelium [18,20].
Both oestrogen (ER) and progesterone (PR) receptors are detectable in luminal epithelial cells using immuno-cytochemical methods [21-23]. In our studies the mean proportion of ER-positive cells was 3.0 ± 3.4% (SD) and of PR-positive cells 11.6 ± 6.8%. Myoepithelial and stromal cells did not stain for either receptor. One or more ER-positive staining cells were seen in 94% of breasts and PR-positive cells were detectable in 100%. However, one or more entirely negative lobules were seen in 44% of breasts with respect to ER and 1.4% for PR. ER declined significantly during the cycle but there was no change in PR expression (Fig. 2). In women taking the oral contraceptive pill (OCP), the decline in ER occurred 1-2 weeks earlier than in natural cycles, suggesting that either oestrogens or progestogens are responsible for down-regulation of ER expression during the cycle. There was little change in the proportion of cells which expressed PR, except for a small rise in the third week during natural cycles.
Thus the epithelium of the breast undergoes marked changes during the cycle. From being rather quiescent in the follicular phase, the luteal phase is associated with increased proliferation, evidence of secretory changes and reduced expression of ER. The appearances can be thought of as a preparation for pregnancy and they return to baseline if fertilisation does not occur.

Changes in the Mesenchyme (Intralobular Stroma) During the Menstrual Cycle

The intralobular stroma of the TDLU was first emphasised by Ozello [24] and further observations were made by Eyden et al. [25]. The intralobular stroma contains several well defined structures which include the basement membrane surrounding the epithelium and a zone of sub-basement membrane connective tissue lying under the attenuated delimiting fibroblasts which completely envelope all the ductules (Fig. 3). Outside the delimiting fibroblasts is a loose association of other fibroblasts, macrophages and lymphocytes, and there is morphological evidence that the fibro-

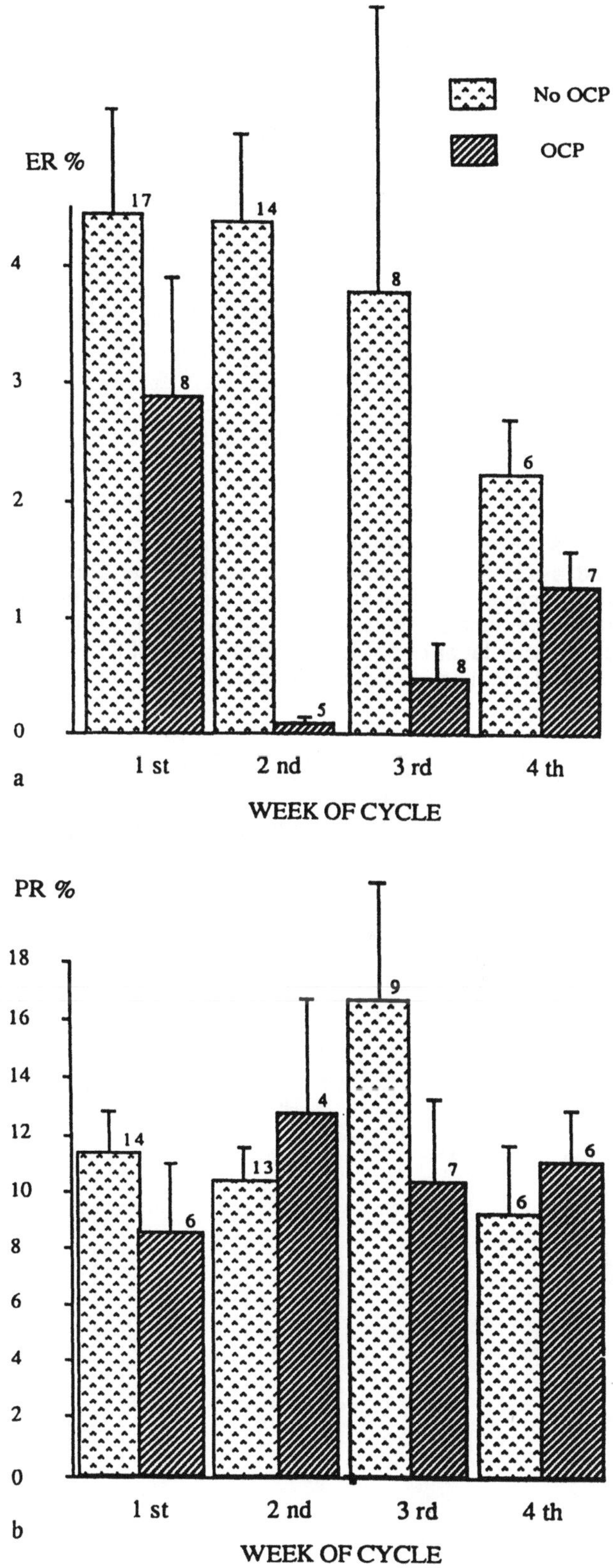

Fig. 2. The proportion of oestrogen receptor-positive and progesterone receptor-positive luminal epithelial cells (mean ± SE) in TDLU in relation to the week of the menstrual cycle and oral contraceptive use

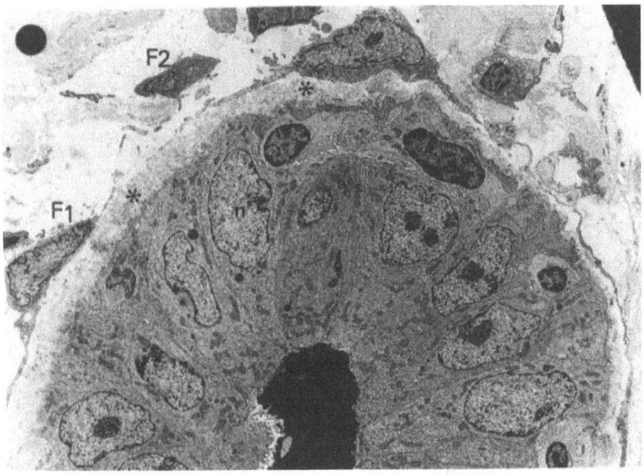

Fig. 3. Electron micrograph of a portion of a ductule and associated intralobular stroma. Luminal epithelial and basal myoepithelial cells are surrounded by dense sub-basement membrane connective tissue (*) below a continuous layer of deliminating fibroblasts (Fl). F2 is a non-deliminating intralobular fibroblast.

blasts form a loose syncytium [24,25]. Lobules are separated from each other by connective tissue with variable density, i.e., the interlobular stroma, which contains a more sparse population of fibroblasts. Specific changes in the appearance and composition of the intralobular stroma have been reported to occur in synchrony with the secretion of ovarian steroid hormones during the menstrual cycle [15,18,24, 26-28].

Recently, we performed a study to determine the distribution of various macromolecular constituents of the intra- and interlobular stroma in the normal breast during the menstrual cycle in order to determine if changes occurred which might indicate that they were under direct or indirect hormonal control. Immunohistochemistry was performed using a panel of polyclonal antibodies to matrix macromolecules and the pattern of staining in relation to the day of the menstrual cycle was estimated (Fig. 4). Rather surprisingly, the expression of collagens type IV and V, heparan sulphate proteoglycan and laminin either diminished or disappeared during the second and third weeks of the menstrual cycle in all the structures of the intralobular stroma, including the basement membrane, sub-basement membrane area and delimiting fibroblasts [28]. This was a specific effect be-

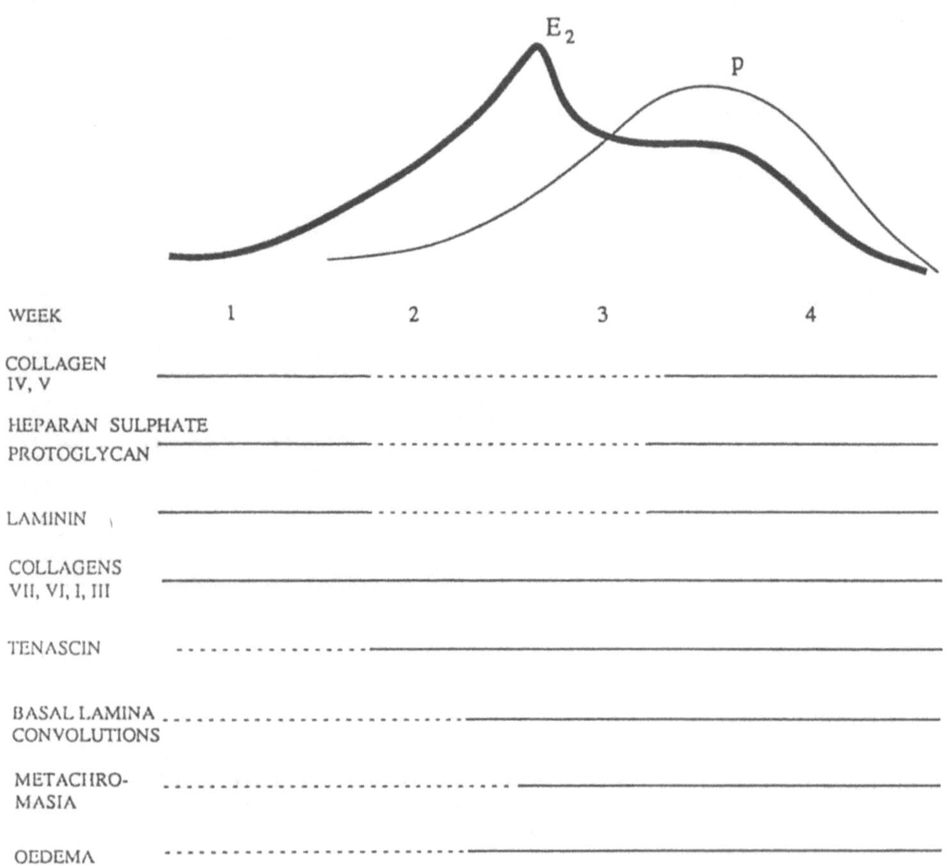

Fig. 4. Summary of change (or lack of changes) in the extracellular matrix in relation to the week of the cycle in relation to changes in serum oestradiol (E2) and progesterone (P). ---------- = reduced expression in comparison to continuous lines.

cause there was no change in staining for collagens I, III, VI and VII and blood vessels within the intralobular stroma which, although containing the same extracellular matrix molecules as the lobular basement membrane, showed no changes during the cycle. These results suggest that the variations observed in the lobule during the cycle reflect hormonally induced changes of extracellular matrix synthesis and/or degradation. Since the changes occur during the period of ovarian oestrogen secretion, it is possible that oestrogen induces enzymes which cause alteration of certain structures in the mesenchyme in preparation for the morphogenic events which take place during pregnancy; in the absence of pregnancy, when oestrogen levels decline at the end of the cycle, the structures are reconstituted.

Tenascin is a novel extracellular matrix glycoprotein which appears to have a major role in cell migration and is increased in foetal and neoplastic tissues. Expression of this molecule is increased in the intralobular stroma during the final two weeks of the cycle [27]. We have also demonstrated markedly increased folding of the basement membrane during this period using electron microscopy [29]. Other groups have demonstrated deposition of metachromatically stained material representing glycosaminoglycans and also oedema of the intralobular stroma occurs during the second half of the cycle [19,26].

Thus, marked changes also occur in many of the connective tissue components of the intralobular stroma during the menstrual cycle, presumably in response to hormonal changes (Fig. 4). As with the epithelium, it is possible that many of these changes can be interpreted as a preparation for expansion of the gland, should pregnancy ensue.

Steroid Control of Cyclical Changes in the TDLU

Breast development and cyclical activity of the breast do not occur in the absence of secretions from the anterior pituitary gland or the ovaries, implying that both steroid and peptide hormones are required for the changes to occur [30]. It is highly likely, as judged by experiments in animals and in *in vitro* experiments using human normal and malignant epithelial cells, that the hormones act, at least partly, by modulating the production and activity of growth factors produced by the epithelial and mesenchymal cells of the TDLU.

The steroid hormones which are candidates for the control of cyclical changes in the TDLU are oestrogen and progesterone since they are produced cyclically by the ovaries. A controversy exists concerning the relative importance of each hormone with respect to the proliferative activity of the luminal epithelial cells of the TDLU during the luteal phase of the cycle. Knowledge of the relative role of each hormone is important with respect to risk and prevention of breast cancer. In the endometrium, where it is clear that proliferation is stimulated by oestrogen, epithelial cell proliferation begins in the mid-follicular phase of the cycle and declines rapidly when rising serum concentrations of progesterone in the early luteal phase inhibit the effect of oestrogen [31]. In contradistinction to the endometrium, breast epithelial cell proliferation is at its minimum at the point of near maximal endometrial proliferation and at its maximum in the mid-luteal phase when the endometrium is non-proliferative (Fig. 5). These findings have led several groups to suggest that progesterone, or a combination of oestrogen and progesterone rather than oestrogen alone, is the major steroid mitogen for the normal mammary epithelium [2,15,32].

The perceived lack of effect of oestrogen alone upon proliferation of the normal breast and reports of lack of an effect of oestrogen upon cell proliferation *in vitro* [33], is at odds with the majority of epidemiological *in vivo* and *in vitro* studies which suggest that oestrogen is a major mitogen for breast epithelium. In order to attempt to resolve this paradox, we implanted biopsies of normal human breast tissue into athymic nude mice with low endogenous oestrogen levels and then assessed the effect of oestrogen and progesterone alone or combined on epithelial cell proliferation by measuring the 3H-thymidine labelling index. Mice were treated with oestrogen and progesterone pellets with differing amounts of hormones in order to produce levels of serum hormones similar to those seen in women at various stages of the menstrual cycle and during pregnancy. The results of some of these experiments are outlined in Figure 6 [34]. Proliferation of the transplanted

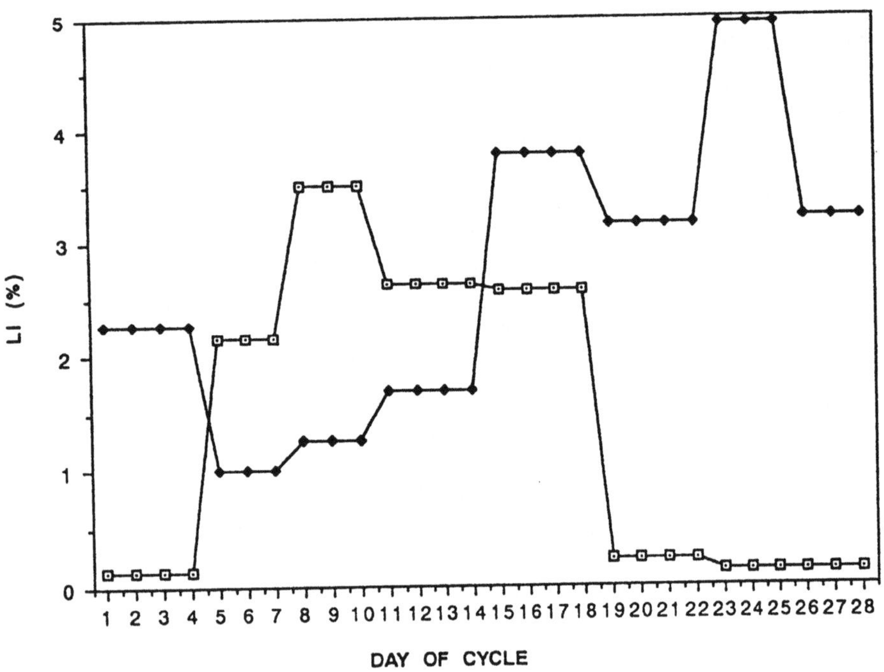

Fig. 5. Thymidine labelling index (LI%) in relation to day of the menstrual cycle in the endometrium (❑) (n=28) after Ferenczy [31] and in the breast (◆) (n=127). The mean of 3-6 day periods was taken for the endometrium by Ferenczy and we have performed the same type of analysis on data derived from normal TDLU. The data are not corrected for age.

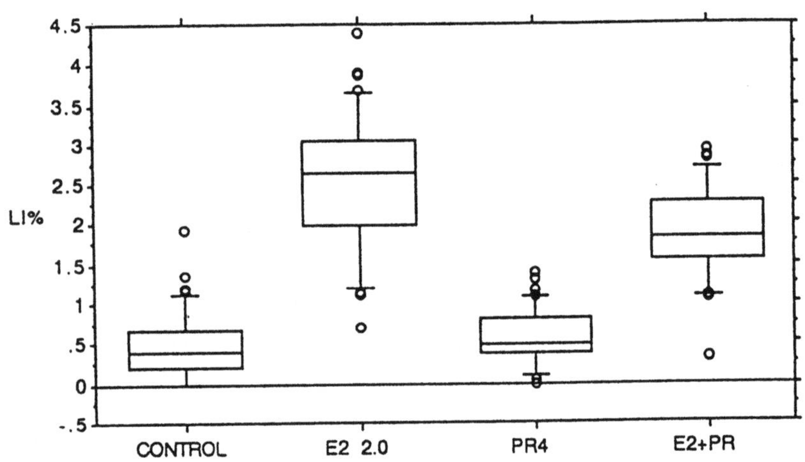

Fig. 6. Thymidine labelling index (LI%) of normal human TDLU implanted into nude mice. Control = no added hormones. E2 2.0 = 2 mg of oestradiol implanted in a silastic pellet; PR4 = pellet with 4 mg of progesterone; E2 + PR = pellets with 2 mg of oestradiol and 4 mg of progesterone.

normal mammary epithelium was stimulated in a dose-dependent manner by oestrogen but not progesterone. A combination of oestrogen and progesterone did not stimulate proliferation more than oestrogen alone. These results of an effect of oestrogen and no, or only a minor effect, of progesterone on epithelial proliferation are in agreement with similar experiments performed by McManus and Welsch [35,36], although the effects of different doses of hormones were not investigated and it is not clear whether they used histologically normal breast tissue.

The differences in peak proliferative activity between the endometrium and the breast during the menstrual cycle may be related to the time course of the need for functional activity of each organ. The endometrium needs to be prepared to receive the fertilised ovum for implantation by the early luteal phase of the cycle, whereas there is no requirement for functional activity of the breast until 9 months later. It is clear from the results of the morphological studies on the breast during the menstrual cycle outlined above that breast lobules vary in their sensitivity to circulating hormones. This variation may have a function in that it would seem inappropriate for all lobules to grow at the same rate to produce, for example, a fully functional breast at the end of the first trimester of pregnancy. The histological appearance of the breast in the second trimester bears out this point since immature and mature lobules exist side by side. Indeed, some primitive lobules do not appear to respond at all to pregnancy since Russo et al. [37] report seeing such structures in near full-term breasts. The physiological basis for the variation in sensitivity of lobules to oestrogen is not known but it may be related to the variation in expression of ER in luminal cells of the TDLUs. It is also possible that variation in lobule and epithelial cell sensitivity may be mediated by mechanisms "distal" to the interactions between the oestradiol/oestrogen receptor complex and its cognate oestrogen response element since it is unlikely (although possible) that ER itself varies in structure throughout the breast. Assessment of the mechanism of the variation in lobule sensitivity within the breast and between subjects is an important goal for future investigation.

The effects of oestrogen and progesterone upon epithelial proliferation are supported by two studies which show that the mid-luteal phase rise in LI is altered by OCP use. Normal breast tissue proliferation was assessed in biopsies obtained from women taking and not taking the OCP [22,38]. In the women taking the OCP the rise in LI which is normally seen in the third week of the natural cycle was seen in the second week (Fig. 7). In addition, a correlation was found between the dose of oestrogen and the LI in the second week, suggesting that oestrogen and not progesterone was the important component of the OCP [38]. However, Anderson et al. [38] also found stimulation of LI during the second week of the cycle in women taking the progestogen-only OCP. This result is surprising in view of the lack of effect of progesterone in the nude mouse experiments described above and could be explained by the relatively small numbers of women studied (n=14) or by the fact that many of the norprogestins used in OCPs have oestrogenic effects in contradistinction to progesterone and its derivatives [39].

We have argued from the nude mouse experiments in particular, that progesterone either does not stimulate or only has a very small stimulatory effect on mammary epithelium. However, Clarke and Sutherland [40] present data showing that progesterone can stimulate

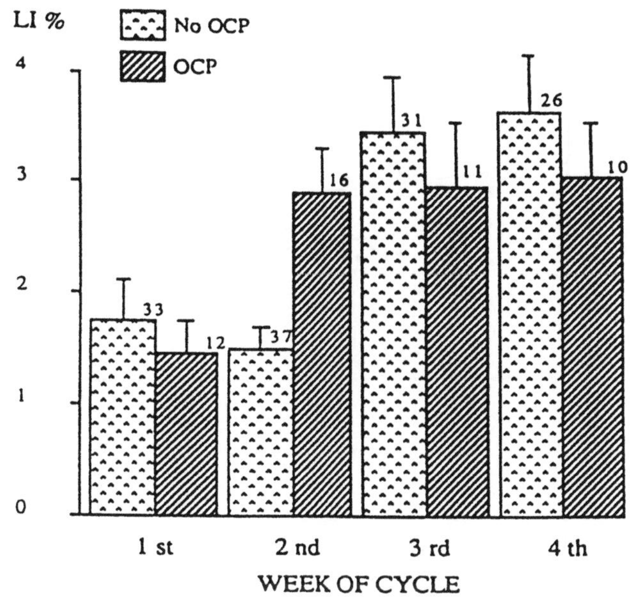

Fig. 7. Thymidine labelling index (LI%, mean ± SE) in relation to week of cycle and OCP use showing a rise in LI during the second week of the cycle in OCP users

epithelial proliferation under physiological conditions. In their extensive review, they conclude that the effect of progesterone is probably transient and may amount to only one cell division. They also point out that, in contrast to the endometrium, progesterone does not appear to have an inhibitory effect on oestrogen-mediated proliferation; this is in agreement with *in-vivo* studies in women and nude mice which indicate that progesterone appears to be largely neutral to mammary epithelial cell proliferation. The changes in the luteal phase of the cycle are consistent with the hypothesis that oestrogen affects cell growth and promotes differentiation [41], whereas progesterone enhances cell function in differentiated cells [42,43].

Oestrogens are also known to stimulate a large number of other cellular functions in addition to proliferation. These include a number of genes for which there is at present no known function (e.g. pS2) and proteases or their precursors, for example, plasminogen activator [44], collagenase type IV [45] and cathepsin D [46]. The apparent loss or diminution of the stromal components from the basement membrane, subbasement region, the delimiting fibroblast and the intralobular stroma during the second and third weeks of the menstrual cycle, which we have demonstrated, could be related to this

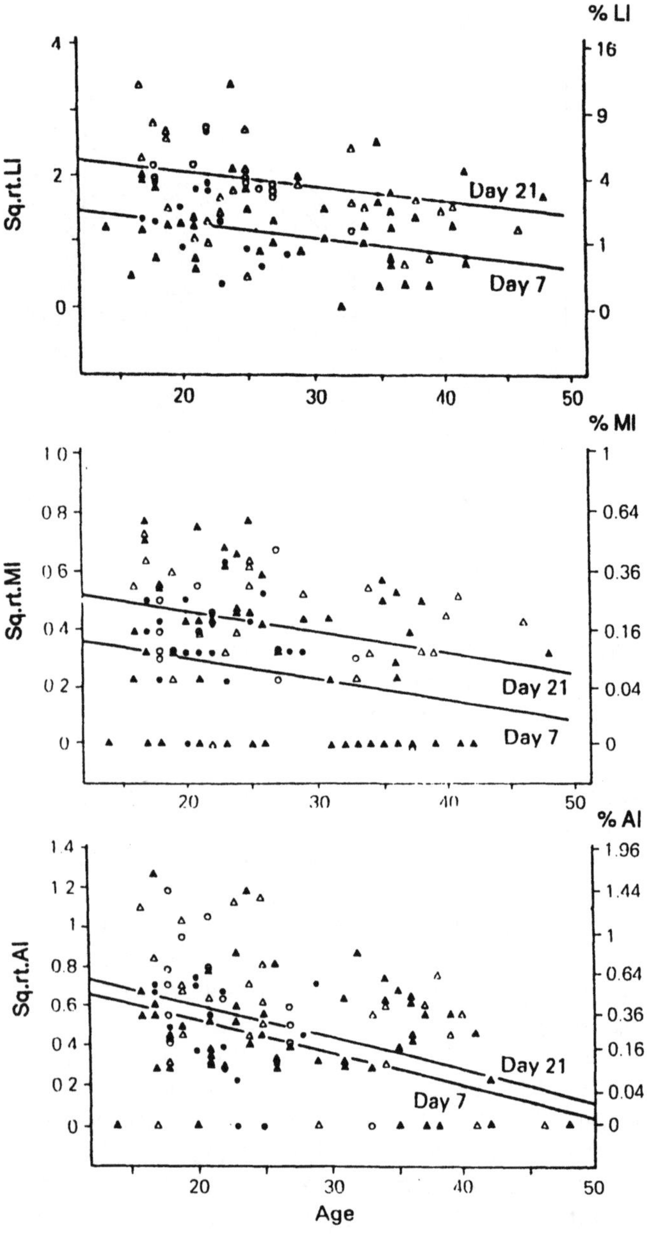

Fig. 8. Decline of LI, MI and apoptotic indices with age. Regression lines indicate fall in indices related to day 7 and 21 of the menstrual cycle. ▲ = first half of cycle off the pill; ● = first half on the pill; △ = second half off the pill; ○ = second half on the pill

effect of oestrogen on the activity of these enzymes. Type IV collagenase has been localised to myoepithelial and epithelial cells of the normal human breast [47]. Oestrogen has also been shown to induce glycosaminoglycan deposition in fibroblasts *in vitro* [48] and in various animals, particularly in the sex skin [49,50]. Oestrogen receptors have not been demonstrated in intralobular fibroblasts from women and it is possible that GAG deposition results from oestrogen stimulation of the synthesis of factors by the epithelial cells which affect intralobular fibroblasts [51].

Changes in the Epithelium with Age

Earlier we described the series of changes which occur in the epithelium and stroma of the TDLU during the menstrual cycle. However, superimposed on this cyclical activity there is evidence that there is a gradual reduction in the amplitude of these changes with increasing age; this phenomenon starts well before the menopause. Changes take place in the epithelium and in the intra- and the extra-lobular stroma and may be regarded as a process of involution of the breast. There is evidence that this process may occur at different rates among individuals.

A decline in labelling index and MI of the epithelium of the TDLU with age has been demonstrated by several groups [12,14,17,37] (Fig. 8). The decline is seen in both halves of the menstrual cycle so that in Figure 8 we have shown regression lines for day 7 and day 21 of the cycle. Although there is an increase in the LI in the luteal phase of the menstrual cycle, this rise occurs later in the older breast, suggesting decreased sensitivity of the epithelium with age (Fig. 9a). The maximum LI is in the third week of the cycle in women aged less than 25 whereas the maximum is in the fourth week in women of 25 years or older. The LI in both the first and second halves of the cycle declines with age, although the biggest change is in the luteal phase where the mean LI falls from 5.5% in women ≤20 to 2.1% in women >30 (Fig. 9b). The age dependence of proliferation is supported by experiments where human mammary epithelium from women of different ages was grown *in vitro*. Fast and slow growing colonies were produced from both young and old women but the fast growing colonies predominated in young women and the slow growing ones in older women [52]. These data support the concept that elevated risk in early reproductive life may be related to the higher rates of cell proliferation during this period [53]. A decline in the apoptotic index occurred in parallel with the decline in MI

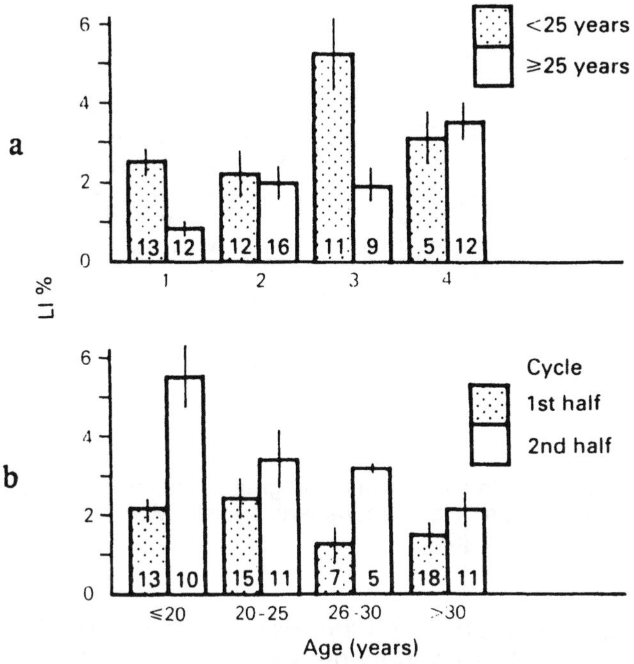

Fig. 9. Labelling index (LI%) of normal epithelium. a) in relation to the week of the menstrual cycle in women <25 yrs and ≥25 years of age; b) in the first and second halves of the cycle in relation to age

and LI, suggesting that the cell production and cell death are reduced in parallel with increasing age (Fig. 8).

Russo et al. [37] carefully dissected the breasts of women who had had reduction mammoplasties in order to determine the types of lobular structures present in relation to age. They concluded that there were 4 morphological types of lobule according to the numbers of ductules (acini) found. Virginal or type I lobules were found predominantly in young women and comprised approximately 11 ductules each (Table 1). Type II and III lobules had more ductules and were found more frequently in older women. Type IV lobules had approximately 180 ductules and were found only in pregnancy. Thymidine labelling studies in the different types of lobule showed the highest labelling index (LI) in type I lobules; the cells of these lobules also concentrated more carcinogen *in vitro* and when dissociated produced more highly proliferative cells than the type II and III lobules [52]. The women who had only type I lobules in their breasts were all nulliparous. Importantly these structures were seen not only in nulliparous women in their late teens but also in nulliparae in their forties, suggesting that a possible reason for the risk of nulliparity is the persistence of highly proliferative virginal lobules and a failure of the breast to age. Russo and Russo [54] argued that the proliferative capacity and sensitivity to carcinogens in humans may parallel that found in animal models where carcinogens were most active in young animals with undifferentiated lobules.

Table 1. DNA labelling index according to the type of lobule [57]

Lobule type	Ductules/lobule	DNA-LI per lobule
I	11.2 ± 6.3	5.4 ± 2.5
II	47.0 ± 11.7	1.0 ± 1.2
III	81.0 ± 16.6	0.2 ± 0.3
IV	180.0 ± 20.0	–

Morphological studies also support a change in the epithelium of the breast with age. Hutson et al. [55] showed that the lobule diameter and volume began to decline in the third decade (Fig. 10). These authors estimated the total amount of epithelial tissue in normal breasts from 58 women who died of non-breast diseases at various ages and showed that the total amount of epithelial tissue declined from a peak of 16% at the age of 30 to 2.5% at the age of 80. The maximum rate of decline was in the premenopausal years. In the postmenopausal period several authors have remarked that epithelial structures of the lobule are often difficult to define.

Changes in the Mesenchyme with Age

Marked changes in the intralobular and interlobular stroma occur with age; these changes, as those seen in the epithelium, begin before the menopause. Hutson et al. [55] estimated the amounts of fibroconnective tissue in lobules and showed a decline from 69% to approximately 60% between the ages of 20 and 60 (Fig. 10). The intralobular tissue becomes more collagenous and less cellular with age until, in the postmenopausal period, it is often difficult to distinguish between the intralobular and extralobular stroma. In contradistinction to the intralobular mesenchyme, Hutson et al. [55]

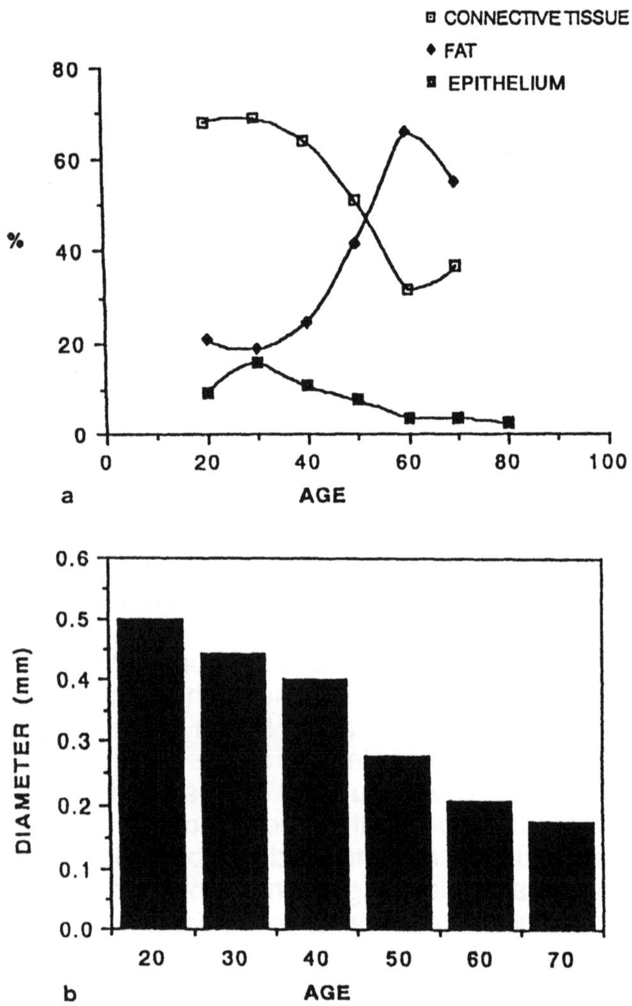

Fig. 10. A: changes in the amount of connective tissue, fat and epithelium in the normal breast with age; B: reduction of mean lobule diameter with age. Modified from Hutson et al. [55]

also reported that the interlobular fibroconnective tissue of the interlobular mesenchyme declines with age and the fat content of the breast increases (Fig. 10).
These well documented effects of age on the intralobular and extralobular mesenchyme in breasts examined postmortem are mirrored by changes in the appearances of mammograms. Brisson et al. [56] evaluated the mammographic parenchymal pattern in a group of 55,053 women in the Breast Cancer Detection Demonstration Project (BCDDP). The patterns were divided into fatty, glandular/dense and intermediate. The proportion of women in each group in relation to age is outlined in Figure 11. These data show the gradual decline of the

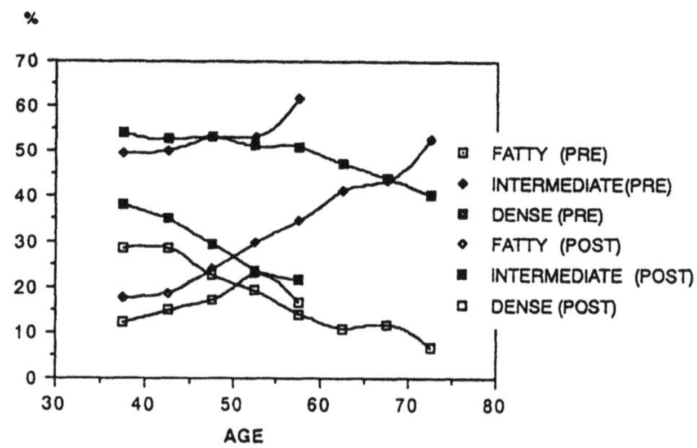

Fig. 11. Changes in mammographic patterns in relation to age and menopausal status. Modified from Brisson et al. [56]

glandular/dense pattern with age from 30-40% at age 40 to approximately 5% at age 70 and an increase of the mammograms described as fatty from approximately 15% to 50% over the same period. The data for pre- and postmenopausal women indicate that the change to a fatty and less dense pattern on the mammogram appears to begin before the menopause and increases at the same rate in premenopausal women as in postmenopausal women of the same age. Thus by direct morphological assessment and indirect mammographic assessment the amount of fibroconnective tissue within the breast appears to decline with age as the breasts increase their fat content. Clearly it is not certain that the mammographic patterns described as fatty or glandular conform to this type of tissue in the breast but histological analysis of breasts after mammography suggests that the dense pattern is associated with areas of dense connective tissue often containing epithelial cells and the "fatty" type of mammogram is associated with an increase in fat tissue [57,58].

The Control of Breast Ageing

Almost all components of the TDLU and the interlobular stroma show gradual changes with increasing age. Any explanation of control mechanisms has to account for the fact that most of the changes begin before the menopause, although they appear to be accelerated by it. Serum oestradiol and IGF-1 levels decline before the menopause and thus may be important controlling factors [59-61]. In addition, epithelial cells derived from TDLUs of older women proliferate less rapidly *in vitro*, suggesting a programmed change in cell sensitivity [52]. If, as we have suggested, the luminal epithelial cell influences the mesenchyme by oestrogen-stimulated paracrine growth factors, the decline in oestradiol levels and possible decreased sensitivity of the cell may lead to a reduction in oestrogen-stimulated events and enhance oestrogen-inhibited events such as the secretion of TGF beta, a growth factor known to be associated with increased fibrosis within the breast [62].

Fibrosis in the interlobular stroma declines with age and this is thought to be responsible for changes in the appearance of mammograms during life. The mechanism of this change is not clear but may also be related to oestrogen. Mammographic patterns tend to remain dense or increase in density in women who take hormone replacement therapy [63,64]. In addition, Huseby and Thomas [65] demonstrated that the interlobular stroma in postmenopausal women taking oestrogen for treatment of advanced breast cancer showed increased numbers and activity of interlobular fibroblasts associated with increased collagen deposition. In this study, oestrogen also reversed changes in the intralobular stroma so that the TDLU reverted to the appearance of the young breast. Oestrogen therefore appears to reduce fibrosis in the intralobular stroma and to increase it in the interlobular stroma. Since oestrogen receptors have not been demonstrated in intralobular fibroblasts, it is difficult to be certain of the mechanism of the oestrogenic effect. However, the differential response to intra- and extralobular fibroblasts may be related to their clonal type since we have demonstrated that the interlobular fibroblasts are foetal in type whereas the intralobular fibroblasts have adult features [66,67].

Summary of Changes Within the Breast

In the introduction we argued that, since most women within a population have similar environments, the variation in risk of breast cancer among individuals may be due to differences in the susceptibility of breasts. Since most breast cancers arise in TDLU, this suggests that the susceptibility of the epithelium or mesenchyme or interactions between the two in these structures are important. Epidemiological and experimental data indicate that the relatively rapidly proliferating epithelium in the young breast is at high risk. The effect of ageing is to reduce the amplitude of proliferation during the cycle and there appears to be a change from type I to type III lobules (a process which may be accelerated by pregnancy).

It is likely that the control of the cyclicity of the epithelium is highly complex and related to the concerted activity of many hormones and growth factors. However, there is strong evidence that the cyclical secretion of oestradiol from the ovaries has a major influence on epithelial proliferation. Since the amplitude of the cycles declines with age, this suggests that the epithelial cells of the TDLU become less sensitive to the proliferative stimulus. The reason for this change is not known but may be partly related to differentiation of lobules from type I to type III; it may also be linked to genetic differences in rates of ageing within TDLU. It is of interest that changes with age, reduction in proliferation, fibrosis of the intralobular stroma and fatty change in the extralobular stroma can be reversed by administration of high doses of oestrogens to postmenopausal women [65]. Fechner [68] reviewed the histological changes in postmenopausal women taking low-dose oestrogens, as given in hormone replacement therapy (HRT), and found no changes in the breasts compared with controls not taking HRT. This suggests that the elderly breast is relatively resistant to oestrogens and may be one reason why HRT does not increase the risk of breast cancer appreciably.

The apparent loss of sensitivity of the TDLU with age (even before the menopause) takes place on a background of marked heterogeneity of responsiveness within any single breast. Proliferating TDLU and non-proliferating TDLU are often seen together. Thus when we hypothesise that some breasts are less sensitive than others, we suggest that the range of sensitivities of TDLU is reduced, implying more quiescent lobules and less proliferative ones rather than an absolute change.

It seems to us likely that the probability of a transforming event in the TDLU is related to the magnitude of the early luteal proliferative response. (It is of interest that the TDLU at this time has some of the features of an *in-situ* or an infiltrating carcinoma, namely proliferation, attenuation of the intralobular stroma, increased GAG synthesis close by, i.e. in the intralobular stroma, and increased fibrosis at a distance, i.e. in the extralobular stroma.) We suggest that the magnitude rather than the duration of proliferation is important since the duration is extended in OCP cycles [22,23] but OCP use is not associated with an appreciable increase in risk of breast cancer [2]. The observations outlined above possibly have implications for the detection of women at risk and the prevention of breast cancer.

Implications for Detection of the Breast at Risk

If the above susceptibility hypothesis is correct, women at risk would be likely to have breasts which are different, albeit quantitatively rather than qualitatively, from those not at risk. Detection of differences among breasts by needle aspiration or biopsy or examination of nipple aspirates would appear to be difficult. Mammographic patterns have already been used to define risk but the sensitivity and specificity of this approach are low [69]. However, if the changes in the breast at risk were more extreme it might be possible to detect them. One approach to testing this hypothesis is to examine the "normal" TDLU in a breast in which an infiltrating carcinoma has been diagnosed. These TDLU might be expected to show differences from TDLU in normal breasts since they may represent an extreme of the normal range of variation of lobules being the type likely to be associated with neoplastic transformation.

Differences in the epithelium and the mesenchyme between normal TDLU in normal breasts and "normal" TDLU in malignant breasts have indeed been reported and are summarised in Table 2. We have assessed L1 and ER expression in TDLU from breasts containing a malignancy and, rather surpris-

Table 2. Documented alterations in morphologically normal lobules in cancer containing breast (compared with lobules from normal breasts)

Feature	Change	Reference
Epithelium		
Apoptosis	Reduced	Allen et al. 1992 [71]
Ultrastructure	Abnormal microvillae	Spring-Mills & Elias 1975 [72]
Cell surface antigens	Unusual expression Increased phenotypic variability	Courtney et al. 1991 [73] Ceriani et al. 1984 [74]
Pentose phosphate shunt activity	Increased	McDermott et al. 1990 [76]
Integrin expression	Reduced alpha B4	Jones et al. 1992 [77]
EGFR and c-*myc*	Increased	Whittaker et al. 1986 [100]
Mesenchyme		
Angiogenesis	Increased	Jensen et al. 1982 [79]
Intralobular fibroblasts	Foetal	Schor et al. 1992 [66]

ingly, have found no differences compared with normal lobules from a normal breast [70]. However, although proliferation in the TDLU does not appear to be increased, we have demonstrated reduced apoptosis in TDLU away from carcinomas which may lead to expansion of an aberrant cell population [71]. Others have shown that the surface of the epithelium changes in that the microvillae become abnormal [72] and surface antigen expression either becomes more like that seen on the adjacent carcinoma [73] or phenotypic variability of antigen expression increases [74]. Many years ago tumours were found to have increased pentose phosphate shunt activity [75] and more recently McDermott et al. [76] demonstrated a similar phenomenon in normal lobules and suggested these biochemical changes may precede the morphological changes of breast carcinogenesis. Jones et al. [77] studied the expression of the alpha-6 and beta-4 subunits of integrins in normal breast lobules from carcinoma breasts and showed reduced reactivity similar to the tumour in 66% of cases, suggesting that loss of these integrins may be an early event in the neoplastic process.

Alterations in normal TDLU in carcinoma containing breasts also appear to affect the mesenchyme. When normal lobules from a malignant breast were transplanted to the rabbit iris, they induced angiogenesis twice as often as lobules from normal breasts [78,79]. Also the intralobular fibroblasts of normal lobules show adult characteristics but normal lobules from malignant breasts contain fibroblasts which have foetal migratory patterns in collagen and secrete a protein we have called migration stimulating factor [66]. Other foetal characteristics have been detected in cancers. Foetal-type collagen [80] and a foetal collagenase [81] have been detected in primary human tumours. Foetal mesenchyme may, in some way, enhance carcinogenesis since implants of foetal mesenchyme in the mammary fat pads of adult mice increased carcinogen-induced tumour development [82].

Thus it appears that many tumours arise on a background of histologically normal lobules which have subtle alterations. These TDLU may represent one end of a spectrum of heterogeneity seen among subjects. Alternatively the lobules could be affected by the tumour in some way. Further studies are required to dissect these possibilities but if the former is true it may be possible to devise assays performed on small biopsies of "normal" tissue in normal breasts which show some of these abnormalities and which may indicate the breast at risk before infiltrating tumours have arisen.

Another almost normal feature (because it is so common) of the normal breast is epithelial hyperplasia. These changes are found in 10-20% of young women; there is a slight drop in frequency around the time of the menopause and then a slow rise with age to approximately 50% of breasts at age 80-90 [83,84]. However, in breasts of premenopausal women which contain a cancer Simpson et al. [85] detected independent areas of hyperplasia in up to 70% of women (Fig. 12), suggesting that a proportion of tumours (approximately 50%) arise from the small group of women with proliferative changes which may be detectable by biopsy and thus indicate risk. Hyperplasia and atypia can be detected on needle aspirations; Skolnik et al. [86] showed that such changes could be detected by 4-quadrant needle aspiration in up to a third of women with ostensibly normal breasts but with a strong family history of breast cancer, although others have failed to find correlations between cytological appearances and subsequent histological examination of biopsies [87].

The data summarised above suggest that many tumours arise on a background of diffuse changes in the TDLU which may be detectable by biopsy. However, perhaps we should inject a word of caution here since there are data which suggest that some tumours arise on a background of widespread changes in the breast and are multicentric and bilateral whereas others appear to arise as a single focus on a background of normality. Data which support this notion are summarised in Table 3. These data are derived from careful studies of breasts ipsilateral and contralateral to *in-situ* or infiltrating tumours where the authors searched assiduously for other foci of tumour using serial sectioning techniques. The data from different studies give remarkably consistent results. About half of all tumours appear to arise in women in whom other independent foci of infiltrating or *in-situ* carcinoma can be found in the same or the contralateral breasts.

It remains to be determined whether any of the changes noted above can be used diagnostically to determine risk in breasts with diffuse

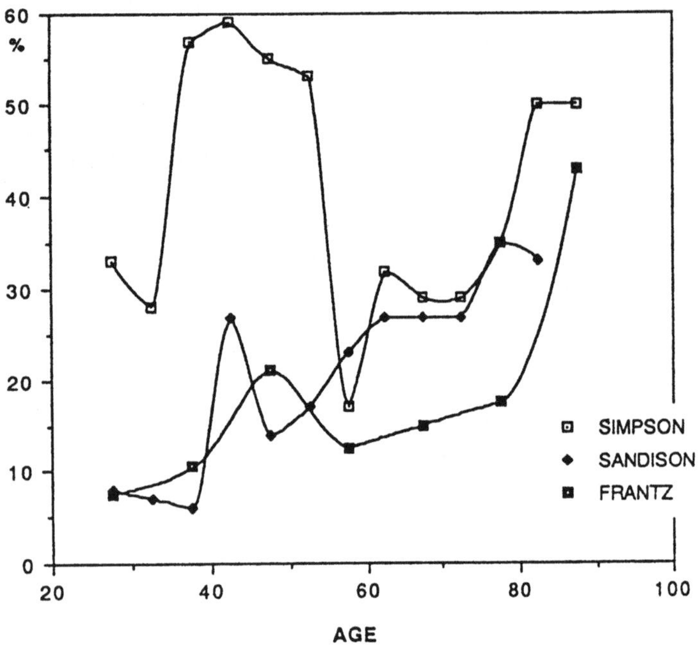

Fig. 12. Proportion of breasts where epithelial hyperplasia was detectable in breasts with [85] and without cancer [83,84]

changes, but such an approach seems worth pursuing.

Implications for Breast Cancer Prevention

The studies on the normal breast outlined earlier in this chapter indicate that a reasonable approach to preventing or reducing breast cancer might be to a) reduce the cyclical activity of the breast, b) increase the rate of ageing, or c) use both of these strategies. Cyclical activity of the breast may be reduced by decreasing the numbers of cycles during reproductive life or by inhibiting the proliferation of the epithelium of the TDLU during the cycle. Bernstein et al. [88] suggested that an achievable preventative strategy might be to reduce the number of cycles by delaying the menarche by appropriate diet or exercise. Pike et al. [89] have proposed that, since an early menopause or bilateral oophorectomy in premenopausal women reduce risk, the same effect may be achieved by inducing an artificial menopause using LHRH agonists. They pro-

Table 3. Incidence of additional *in-situ* or infiltrating carcinomas in other quadrants of cancer containing breasts (multicentricity) or in the contralateral breast (bilaterality)

Author	Multicentricity	(%)	Bilaterality	(%)	Author
Alpers & Wellings 1984 [101]	33 of 63	(52)	30 of 63	(48)	Alpers & Wellings 1984 [101]
Ringberg et al. 1991 [102]	39 of 52	(75)	25 of 52	(48)	Ringberg et al. 1991 [102]
Schwartz et al. 1980 [103]	19 of 44	(44)	57 of 84	(68)	Nielsen et al. 1986 [109]
Cahill et al. 1983 [104]	91 of 186	(49)			
Sarnelli & Squartini 1989 [105]	31 of 67	(47)	112 of 199	(56)	**Total**
Egan 1982 [106]	71 of 118	(60)			
Anastassiades et al. 1993 [107]	183 of 366	(50)			
Qualheim & Gall 1956 [108]	85 of 157	(54)			
Total	552 of 1053	(52)			

posed also that the harmful effects of ovarian ablation, in particular the increased risk of coronary heart disease and osteoporosis, could be reversed by "low dose" oestrogen replacement therapy sufficient to maintain bone density and diminish lipid levels but insufficient to stimulate epithelial proliferation in the TDLU. The harmful effects of continuous oestradiol on the endometrium could be prevented by intermittent "low dose" progestogens. A trial of this approach is in progress in Los Angeles and as an early surrogate endpoint there has been a significant reduction in mammographic density in the treated group compared with untreated control women [90].

Trials of direct inhibition of mammary epithelial cell proliferation (and of premalignant and early malignant lesions) using the antioestrogen tamoxifen are in progress in the USA, Europe and Australasia. The rationale of the use of tamoxifen are the observations that carcinogen-induced mammary tumour formation is inhibited in rodent models [91] and that the incidence of contralateral tumours is reduced in women given adjuvant tamoxifen for early breast cancer. Tamoxifen trials are being performed in women at high risk by virtue, mainly, of a strong family history and in older women because of the increased risk with age. Second-generation anti-oestrogens may be even more effective.

Another approach to prevention might be to increase the rate of ageing or differentiation of the breast. The observation that pregnancy is protective in women and in carcinogen-induced animal tumour models leads to the suggestion that a pseudopregnancy induced by steroids or other hormones should be considered as a possible preventative strategy. Several groups have shown that treatment of rats with the oral contraceptive combination of norethynodrel-mestranol (Enovid) prevents DMBA-induced carcinogenesis [92-94]. Russo et al. [94] demonstrated that human chorionic gonadotrophin (HCG) is also effective in preventing DMBA-induced tumours; HCG induced gland differentiation, reduced the proliferative activity of the epithelium, reduced binding of DMBA to DNA and increased the DNA repair capability of the epithelium. The mechanism of action of HCG is not clear but it may act via the ovary or may directly inhibit epithelial proliferation. Whether treatment with HCG would be effective in women at risk is not known.

Alternative ways of inhibiting proliferation and stimulating differentiation may be by the use of retinoids (in clinical trial in Italy) and non-hypercalcaemic vitamin D analogues (which are known to inhibit the proliferation of established tumours). Other approaches include use of the monoterpioids such as limonene, which have a multiplicity of potentially beneficial activities on the mammary gland [95].

Summary and Conclusions

In this review we have summarised data concerning the changes in the human breast which occur during the menstrual cycle and with increasing age in the epithelium and in the mesenchyme of the TDLU. We have suggested that the highly proliferative epithelium of the TDLU during the luteal phase of the cycle may predispose to malignancy and may account for the epidemiological data which indicates that young breasts are more sensitive to carcinogenesis. A decrease in the rate at which the breast ages may maintain it in a relatively highly proliferative state which may also enhance risk.

Epithelial proliferation in the TDLU is influenced by peptide and steroid hormones and growth factors. However, we have summarised evidence that oestrogen is of central importance in stimulating proliferation. The wide variation in the proliferative activity between breasts, and possibly in the rates of ageing, may be related to variation in sensitivity of the TDLU to oestrogen. Increased chance of neoplasia may be related to reduced time for DNA repair [52] and increased DNA adduct formation [96] in oestrogen-stimulated highly proliferative epithelium. The increased cell proliferation model of carcinogenesis [97] is attractive in the context of the breast; however, it has been pointed out that this may be an oversimplification of the carcinogenic process [98].

A corollary of the breast sensitivity hypothesis is that it may be possible to detect diagnostic changes in the breast at risk and this supposition is supported by the series of alterations detected in lobules from breasts containing a carcinoma compared with lobules from non-neoplastic breasts described here. In addition it may be possible to determine risk by measuring the products of the at-risk epithelium or mesenchyme in serum [99]. Detection of the breast at risk is becoming increasingly important in the context of chemoprevention and mammographic screening programmes.

Finally we discussed the possibilities for prevention based on inhibition of the cyclical activity or an increase in the rate of ageing or differentiation of the breast. A number of chemoprevention trials are in progress and it should be possible to devise other approaches to be tested. Because the results of these trials will take many years to complete, there is a need to devise surrogate endpoints which will give an indication of the effect of a particular chemopreventive agent on the breast. It should be possible to devise endpoints based on our knowledge of the changes which occur in the breast with age and during the menstrual cycle.

REFERENCES

1 Kelsey JL, Berkowitz GS: Breast cancer epidemiology. Cancer Res 1988 (48): 5615-5623

2 Key TJA and Pike MC: The role of oestrogens and progestagens in the epidemiology and prevention of breast cancer. Eur J Cancer Clin Onc 1988 (24):29-43

3 DeWaard F and Trichopoulos D: A unifying concept of the aetiology of breast cancer. Int J Cancer 1988 (41):666-669

4 Willett WC, Stampfer MJ, Colditz GA, Rosner BA, Hennekens CH and Speizer FE: Dietary fat and the risk of breast cancer. New Engl J Med 1987 (316):22-28

5 Boyd NF, Martin LJ, Noffel M, Lockwood GA and Tritchler DL: A meta-analysis of studies of dietary fat and breast cancer risk. Br J Cancer 1993 (68):627-636

6 Hall JM, Lee MK, Newman B, Morrow JE, Anderson LA: Linkage of early-onset familial breast cancer to chromosome 17q21. Science 1990 (250):1684-1689

7 Wellings SR, Jensen HM and Marcum RG: An atlas of subgross pathology of the human breast with special reference to possible precancerous lesions. JNCI 1975 (55): 231-273

8 Kratochwil K: In vitro analysis of the hormonal basis for the sexual dimorphism in the embryonic development of the mouse mammary gland. J Embryol Exp Morph 1971 (25):141-153

9 Sakakura T: New aspects of stroma-parenchyma relations in mammary gland differentiation. Int Rev Cytology 1991 (125):165-201

10 Henderson BE, Ross RK, Judd HL, Krailo MD and Pike MC: Do regular ovulatory cycles increase breast cancer risk? Cancer 1985 (56):1206-1208

11 Pike MC, Krailo MD, Henderson BE, Casagrande JT and Hoel DG: 'Hormonal', risk factors, 'breast tissue age' and the age-incidence of breast cancer. Nature 1983 (303):767

12 Meyer JS: Cell proliferation in normal human breast ducts, fibroadenomas, and other ductal hyperplasia measured by nuclear labelling with tritiated thymidine. Effects of menstrual phase, age, and oral contraceptive hormones. Human Pathol 1977 (8):57

13 Masters JRW, Drife JO, Scarisbrick JJ: Cyclic variation of DNA synthesis in human breast epithelium. JNCI 1977 (58): 1263

14 Anderson TJ, Ferguson DJP and Raab GM: Cell turnover in the "resting" human breast: influence of parity, contraceptive pill, age and laterality. Br J Cancer 1982 (46): 376-382

15 Longacre TA and Bartow SA: A correlative morphologic study of human breast and endometrium in the menstrual cycle. Am J Surg Path 1986 (10):382-393

16 Going JJ, Anderson TJ Battersby S and Macintyre CCA: Proliferative and secretory activity in human breast during natural and artificial menstrual cycles. Am J Path 1988 (130):193-204

17 Potten CS, Watson RJ, Williams GT, Tickle S, Roberts SA, Harris M and Howell A: The effect of age and menstrual cycle upon proliferative activity of the normal human breast. Br J Cancer 1988 (58):163-170

18 Fanger H and Ree HJ: Cyclic changes of human mammary gland epithelium in relation to the menstrual cycle - an ultrastructural study. Cancer 1974 (34): 574-585

19 Vogel PM, Georgiade NG, Fetter BF, Vogel FS and McCarty KS: The correlation of histologic changes in the human breast with the menstrual cycle. Am J Pathol 1981 (104):23-34

20 Ahmed A: Atlas of the ultrastructure of human breast diseases. Churchill Livingstone, Edinburgh 1978

21 Markopoulos C, Berger U, Wilson P, Gazet J-C and Coombes RC: Oestrogen receptor content of normal breast cells and breast carcinomas throughout the menstrual cycle. Br Med J 1988 (296):1349-1351

22 Williams G, Anderson E, Howell A, Watson R, Coyne J, Roberts SA and Potten C: Oral contraceptive use increases proliferation and decreases oestrogen receptor content of epithelial cells in the normal human breast. Int J Cancer 1991 (48):206-210

23 Battersby S, Robertson BJ, Anderson TJ, King RJ and McPherson K: Influence of menstrual cycle, parity and oral contraceptive use on steroid hormone receptors in normal breast. Br J Cancer 1992 (65):601-607

24 Ozzello L: Epithelial-stromal junction of normal and dysplastic mammary glands. Cancer 1970 (25):586-600

25 Eyden BP, Watson RJ, Harris M and Howell A: Intralobular stromal fibroblasts in the resting human mammary gland: ultrastructural properties and intercellular relationships. J Submicrosc Cytol 1986 (18):397-408

26 Ozzello L and Speer FD: The mucopolysaccharides in the normal and diseased breast. Their distribution and significance. Am J Pathol 1958 (34):993-1009

27 Ferguson JE, Schor AM, Howell A and Ferguson MWJ: Tenascin distribution in the normal human breast is altered during the menstrual cycle and in carcinoma. Differentiation 1990 (42): 199-207

28 Ferguson JE, Schor AM, Howell A and Ferguson MWJ: Changes in the extracellular matrix of the normal human breast during the menstrual cycle. Cell and Tissue Res 1992 (268): 167-177

29 Watson RJ, Eyden BP, Howell A and Sellwood RA: Ultrastructural observations on the basal lamina in the normal human breast. J Anat 1988 (156): 1-10

30 Howell A: Clinical evidence for the involvement of oestrogen in the development and progression of breast cancer. Proc Roy Soc Edinburgh 1989 (95B):49-57

31 Ferenczy A, Bertrand G and Gelfand MM: Proliferation kinetics of human endometrium during the nornal menstrual cycle. Am J Obstet Gynecol 1978 (133): 859-867

32 Ferguson DJP and Anderson TJ: Morphological evaluation of cell turnover in relation to the menstrual cycle in the "resting" human breast. Br J Cancer 1981 (44):177-181

33 Yang J, Larson L, Flynn D, Elias J and Nandi S: Serum free primary culture of human normal mammary epithelial cells in collagen gel matrix. Cell Biol Inter Rep 1982 (6):969-975

34 Laidlaw ID: MD Thesis. University of Newcastle 1993

35 McManus MJ and Welsch CW: Hormone-induced ductal DNA synthesis of human breast tissues maintained in the athymic nude mouse. Cancer Research 1981 (41): 3300-3305

36 McManus MJ and Welsch CW: The effect of estrogen, progesterone, thyroxine, and human placental lactogen on DNA synthesis of human breast ductal epithelium maintained in athymic nude mice. Cancer 1984 (54): 1920-1927

37 Russo J, Calaf G, Roi L, Russo IH: Influence of age and gland topography on cell kinetics of normal breast tissue. JNCI 1987 (78): 413

38 Anderson TJ, Battersby S. King RJB, McPherson K and Going JJ: Oral contraceptive use influences resting breast proliferation. Human Pathology 1989 (20): 1139-1144

39 Catherino WH, Jeng MH and Jordan VC: Norgestrel and gestodene stimulate breast cancer cell growth through an oestrogen receptor mediated mechanism. Br J Cancer 1993 (67):945-952

40 Clarke CL and Sutherland RL: Progestin regulation of cellular proliferation. Endocrine Reviews 1990 (11): 266-301

41 Kohler PO, Grimley PM and O'Malley BW: Estrogen-induced cytodifferentiation of the ovalbumin-secreting glands of the chick oviduct. J Cell Biol 1969 (40): 8-27

42 Oka T and Schimke RT: Interaction of estrogen and progesterone in chick oviduct development - II. Effects of estrogen and progesterone on tubular gland cell function. J Cell Biol 1969 (43):123-137

43 O'Malley BW and McGuire WL: Studies on the mechanism of action of progesterone in regulation of the synthesis of specific protein. J Clin Invest 1968 (47): 654-664

44 Butler WB, Kirkland WL, Jorgenson TL: Induction of plasminogen activator by estrogen in a human breast cancer cell line MCF-7. BBRC 1979 (90):1328-1334

45 Shafie SM and Liotta LA: Formation of metastasis by human breast carcinoma cells in nude mice. Cancer Lett 1980 (11):81-87

46 Rochefort H, Augereau P: Structure, function, regulation and clinical significance of the 52K procathepsin D secreted by breast cancer cells. Biochimie 1988 (70):943-949

47 Montiagndo C, Merino MJ, San Juan J, Liotta LA and Stetler-Stevenson WG: Immunihistochemical distribution of type IV collagenase in normal, benign and malignant breast tissue. Am J Pathol 1990 (136): 585-592

48 Ozzello L and Bembry JY: Effects of 17ß oestradiol on the production of acid mucopolysaccharides by cell cultures of human fibroblasts. Nature 1964 (203):80-81

49 Asboe-Hanson G: Hormonal effects on connective tissue. Physiol Rev 1958 (38): 446-462

50 Ogston AG, Philpot JSL, Zuckerman S: Observations related to the swelling of sexual skin in rhesus monkeys. J Endocrinol 1939 (1):231-238

51 Kataoka H, DeCastro R, Zucker S and Biswas C: Tumor cell-derived collagenase-stimulatory factor increases expression of interstitial collagenase, stromelysin and 72-kDa gelatinase. Cancer Res 1993(53):3154-3158

52 Russo J and Russo IH: Biological and molecular bases of mammary carcinogenesis. Lab Invest 1987 (57):112-137

53 Albanes D and Winick M: Are cell number and cell proliferation risk factors for cancer? JNCI 1988 (80): 772-775

54 Russo J and Russo IH: Role of differentiation on transformation of human breast epithelial cells. In: Medina D, Kidwell W, Heppner G and Anderson E (eds) Cellular and Molecular Biology of Mammary Cancer. Plenum Press, New York 1987 pp 399-417

55 Hutson SW, Cowen PN and Bird CC: Morphometric studies of age-related changes in normal human breast and their significance for evolution of mammary cancer. J Clin Path 1985 (38): 281-287

56 Brisson J, Morrison AS and Khalid N: Mammographic parenchymal features and breast cancer in the breast cancer detection demonstration project. JNCI 1988 (80): 1534-1540

57 Arthur JE, Ellis IO, Flowers C, Roebuck E, Elston CW and Blamey RW: The relationship of "high risk" mammographic patterns to histological risk factors for development of cancer in the human breast. Br J Radiol 1990 (63):845-849

58 Wellings SR and Wolfe JN: Correlative studies of the histological and radiographic appearance of the breast parenchyma. Radiology 1978 (129):299-306

59 MacMahon B, Cole P, Brown JB: Oestrogen profiles of Asian and North American women. Lancet 1971 (ii):900-902

60 Apter D, Reinila M and Vihko R: Some endocrine characteristics of early menarche, a risk factor for breast cancer, are preserved into adulthood. Int J Cancer 1989 (44):783-787

61 Peyrat JP, Bonneterre J, Hecquet B, Vennin P, Louchez MM, Fournier C, Lefebvre J and Demaille A: Plasma insulin-like growth factor-1 (IGF-1) concentrations in human breast cancer. Eur J Cancer 1993 (29A): 492-497

62 Silberstein GB, Strickland P, Coleman S and Daniel CW: Epithelium-dependent extracellular matrix synthesis in transforming growth factor-ß1-growth-inhibited mouse mammary gland. J Cell Biol 1990 (110):2209-2219

63 Berkowitz JE, Gatewood OMB, Goldblum LE and Gayler BW: Hormonal replacement therapy: mammographic manifestations. Radiology 1990 (174):199-201

64 Stomper PC, Van Voorhis BJ, Ravnikar VA and Meyer JE: Mammographic changes associated with postmenopausal hormone replacement therapy: A longitudinal study. Radiology 1990 (174): 487-490

65 Huseby RA and Thomas LB: Histological and histochemical alterations in the normal breast tissues of patients with advanced breast cancer

being treated with oestrogenic hormones. Cancer 1954 (7):54-61
66 Schor AM, Schor SL, Ferguson JE, Rushton G, Howell A and Ferguson MWJ: Heterogeneity in the stromal components of the mammary gland: relevance to the development of breast disease. In: Mansel RE (ed) Benign Breast Disease. Parthenon Publishing Gp, Carnforth 1992 pp 115-129
67 Schor SL, Grey AM, Ellis I, Schor AM, Howell A, Sloan P and Murphy R: Fetal-like fibroblasts: their production of migration stimulating factor and role in tumour progression. In: Lippman M and Dickson R (eds) The Molecular and Cell Biology of Breast Cancer (in press)
68 Fechner RE: Benign breast disease in women on estrogen therapy. Cancer 1972 (29): 273-279
69 Saftlas AF and Szklo M: Mammographic parenchymal patterns and breast cancer risk. Epidemiol Rev 1987 (9): 146-174
70 Williams GT, Anderson E, Watson RJ, Coyne J, Roberts SA, Potten CS and Howell A: A comparative study of indices of cell proliferation and the expression of oestrogen and progesterone receptors in lobules of the normal breast tissue adjacent to fibroadenoma or carcinoma. 1993 (in preparation)
71 Allan DJ, Howell A, Roberts SA, Williams GT, Watson RJ, Coyne JD, Clarke RB, Laidlaw IJ and Potten CS: Reduction in apoptosis relative to mitosis in histologically normal epithelium accompanies fibrocystic change and carcinoma of the premenopausal human breast. J Path 1992 (167):25-32
72 Spring-Mills E and Elias JL: Cell surface differences in ducts from cancerous and non-cancerous breasts. Science 1975 (188): 947-949
73 Courtney FP, Williams S and Mansel RE: Monoclonal antibody 323/A3, an indicator for the presence of breast carcinoma. Cancer Lett 1991 (57):115-119
74 Ceriani RL, Peterson JA and Blank EW: Variability in surface antigen expression of human breast epithelial cells cultured from normal breast, normal tissue peripheral to breast carcinomas and breast carcinomas. Cancer Res 1984 (44):3033-3039
75 Weber G: Enzymology of cancer cells. New Engl J Med 1977 (297):486-493
76 McDermott EWM, Barron ET, Smyth PPA and O'Higgins NJ: Premorphological metabolic changes in human breast carcinogenesis. Br J Surg 1990 (77): 1179-1182
77 Jones JL, Critchley DR and Walker RA: Alteration of stromal protein and integrin expression in breast - a marker of premalignant change? J Pathol 1992 (167): 399-406
78 Brem SS, Jenson HM and Gullino PM: Angiogenesis as a marker of preneoplastic lesions of the human breast. Cancer 1978 (41):239-244
79 Jensen HM, Chen I, DeVault MR and Lewis AE: Angiogenesis induced by "normal" human breast tissue: A probable marker for precancer. Science 1982 (218):293-295
80 Pucciminafra I, Luparello C, Andriolo M, Basirico L, Aquino A and Minafra S: A new form of tumor and foetal collagen that binds laminin. Biochem 1993 (32):7421-7427
81 Basset P, Bellocq JP, Wolf C, Stoll I, Hutin P, Limacher JM, Podhajcer OL, Chenard MP, Rio MC and Chambon P: A novel metalloproteinase gene specifically expressed in stromal cells of breast carcinomas. Nature 1990 (348): 699-704
82 Sakakura T, Sakagami Y and Nishizuka Y: Acceleration of mammary cancer development by grafting of fetal mammary mesenchymes in C3H mice. Gan 1979 (70): 459-466
83 Frantz VK, Pickren JW, Melcher GW, Auchincloss H: Incidence of chronic cystic disease in so-called "normal breasts". Cancer 1954 (4):762-783
84 Sandison AT: An autopsy study of the adult human breast. NCI Monograph 1962 (4):1
85 Simpson HW, Mutch F, Halberg F, Griffiths K and Wilson D: Bimodal age-frequency distribution of epitheliosis in cancer mastectomies. Cancer 1982 (50):2417-2422
86 Skolnick MH, Cannon-Albright LA, Goldgar DE, Ward JH, Marshall CJ, Schumann GB, Hogle H, McWhorter WP, Wright EC, Tran TD, Bishop DT, Kushner JP and Eyre HJ: Inheritance of proliferative breast disease in breast cancer kindreds. Science 1990 (250):1715-1720
87 Stanley MW, Henry-Stanley MJ and Zera R: Atypia in breast fine-needle aspiration smears correlates poorly with the presence of a prognostically significant proliferative lesion of a ductal epithelium. Human Path 1993 (24):630-635
88 Bernstein L, Ross RK, Lobo R, Hanisch R, Krailo MD and Henderson BE: The effects of moderate physical activity on menstrual cycle patterns in adolescence: implications for breast cancer prevention. Br J Cancer 1987 (55): 681
89 Pike MC, Ross RK, Lobo RA, Key TJA, Potts M and Henderson BE: LHRH agonists and the prevention of breast and ovarian cancer. Br J Cancer 1989 (60): 142-148
90 Pike MC: Personal communication
91 Jordan VC, Lababidi MK and Langan-Fahey: Suppression of mouse mammary tumorigenesis by long-term tamoxifen therapy. JNCI 1991(83): 492-496
92 Russo IH and Russo J: Hormone prevention of mammary carcinogenesis: A new approach in anticancer research. Anticancer Res 1988 (8): 1247-1264
93 Russo IH, Koszalka M and Russo J: Human chorionic gonadtrophin and rat mammary cancer prevention. JNCI 1990 (82):1286-1289
94 Russo IH, Koszalka M and Russo J: Comparative study of the influence of pregnancy and hormonal treatment on mammary carcinogenesis. Br J Cancer 1991 (64): 481-484
95 Gould MN, Wacker WD and Maltzman TH: Chemoprevention and chemotherapy of mammary tumors by monoterpenoids. In: Pariza MW, Aeschbacker H-U, Felton JS and Sato S (eds) Mutagens and Carcinogens in the Diet. Wiley-Liss Inc, New York 1990 pp 255-268
96 Zaidi SNH, Laidlaw I, Howell A, Potten CS and O'Connor PJ: Normal human breast xenografts activate N-nitroso-dimethylamine: Identification of

potential target cells for an environmental nitrosamine. Br J Cancer 1992 (66):79-83
97 Preston-Martin S, Pike MC, Ross RK, Henderson BE: Epidemiologic evidence for the increased cell proliferation model of carcinogenesis. In: Butterworth B, Slaga T, Farland W and McCain M (eds) Chemically Induced Cell Proliferation: Implications for Risk Assessment. Wiley-Liss Inc, New York 1991 pp 21-34
98 Weinstein IB: Mitogenesis is only one factor in carcinogenesis. Science 1991 (251): 387-388
99 Picardo M, Schor SL, Grey A-M, Howell A, Laidlaw I, Redford J and Schor AM: Migration stimulating activity in serum of breast cancer patients. Lancet 1991 (337):130-133
100 Whittaker J, Walker RA and Varley JM: Differential expression of cellular oncogenes in benign and malignant human breast tissue. In J Cancer 1986 (38):651-655
101 Alpers CE and Wellings SR: The prevalence of carcinoma in situ in normal and cancer associated breasts. Hum Pathol 1985 (16): 796-807
102 Ringberg A, Palmer B, Linell F, Rychterova V and Ljungberg O: Bilateral and multifocal breast carcinoma. A clinical and autopsy study with special emphasis on carcinoma in situ. Eur J Surg Onc 1991 (17):20-29
103 Schwartz GF, Patchesfsky AS, Feig SA, Shaber GS and Schwartz AB: Multicentricity of non-palpable breast cancer. Cancer 1980 (45):2913-2916
104 Cahill CJ, Gibbs NM, Boulter PS, Brient MJ and Price JL: Invasive breast cancer - the tip of an iceberg. Ann Roy Coll Surg England 1983 (65): 356-359
105 Sarnelli R and Squartini F: Cancerous versus noncancerous breasts. Virchows Archiv A Pathol Anat 1989 (414): 257-262
106 Egan RL: Multicentric breast carcinomas: Clinical-radiographic-pathologic whole organ studies and 10 year survival. Cancer 1982 (49):1123-1130
107 Anastassiades O, Iakovou E, Stavridou N, Gogas J and Karameris A: Multicentricity in breast cancer. A study of 366 cases. Am J Clin Pathol 1993 (99):238-243
108 Qualheim RE and Gall EA: Breast carcinoma with multiple sites of origin. Cancer 1957 (10):460-468
109 Nielsen M, Christensen L and Andersen J: Contralateral cancerous breast lesions in women with clinical invasive breast carcinoma. Cancer 1986 (57): 897-903

Inhibition of Oestrogen Receptor Function by Antioestrogens

Malcolm G. Parker

Laboratory of Molecular Endocrinology, Imperial Cancer Research Fund, Lincoln's Inn Fields, London WC2A 3PX, United Kingdom

The importance of endocrine therapy for the treatment of breast cancer has been recognised for almost a century following the pioneering work of Beatson. In advanced disease the most commonly used first-line endocrine therapy is antioestrogen treatment with the non-steroidal antagonist tamoxifen and this has recently also become established in adjuvant therapy after removal of the primary tumour [1,2]. The success of tamoxifen as a therapeutic antioestrogen results, in part, because it is accompanied by beneficial side effects which appear to arise from partial agonistic activity of the drug. These effects include the maintenance of bone density [3,4] and the reduction in blood cholesterol levels which may lead to reduced mortality due to coronary heart disease [5,6].

In spite of the efficacy of tamoxifen treatment most patients eventually develop drug resistance. Oestrogens acting through the oestrogen receptor still seem to be involved since as many as one-half of these patients respond to alternative forms of endocrine therapy. For example, aromatase inhibitors to block oestradiol production are commonly used as a second-line endocrine therapy. Another possibility is the use of alternative antioestrogens, providing their mechanism of action differs from that of tamoxifen. One of these, ICI 182,780, which was developed as a "pure" antioestrogen lacking any agonist activity, is being clinically evaluated at the moment.

The purpose of this chapter is to outline what is currently known about the structure and function of the oestrogen receptor and to describe the molecular mechanism of action of the antioestrogens tamoxifen and, in particular, ICI 182,780. In addition, unresolved problems such as tamoxifen resistance and the molecular basis for the agonistic activity of antioestrogens will be discussed.

Mechanism of Action of Oestrogens

Oestrogen action is mediated by soluble receptors located predominantly in the nucleus of target cells [7]. Upon hormone binding, the oestrogen receptor functions directly as a transcription factor to regulate the transcription of specific genes [8]. The human protein contains 599 amino acids and is made up of 3 discrete structural domains (Fig. 1). The C-terminal domain from residue ~310 is responsible for oestrogen binding but also plays a role in dimerisation and transcriptional activation. Residues 180-310 are responsible for DNA binding and nuclear localisation while the third domain comprising N-terminal 180 residues contains a second transcriptional activation region. Ligand binding is essential to promote receptor dimerisation, high affinity DNA binding and optimum transcriptional activation (Fig. 2).

Individual residues throughout the hormone binding domain appear to be required for high affinity binding of both oestrogens and antioestrogens. The first approach to identify important residues was to affinity label the receptor with synthetic ligands. In the human oestrogen receptor a cysteine at position 530 towards the C-terminus of the protein (equivalent to 534 in the mouse receptor) was affinity labelled with both an oestrogen, ketononestrol aziridine, and an antioestrogen, tamoxifen aziridine, suggesting that this residue is in the vicinity of the ligand binding pocket [9]. This cysteine residue itself is unlikely to be involved

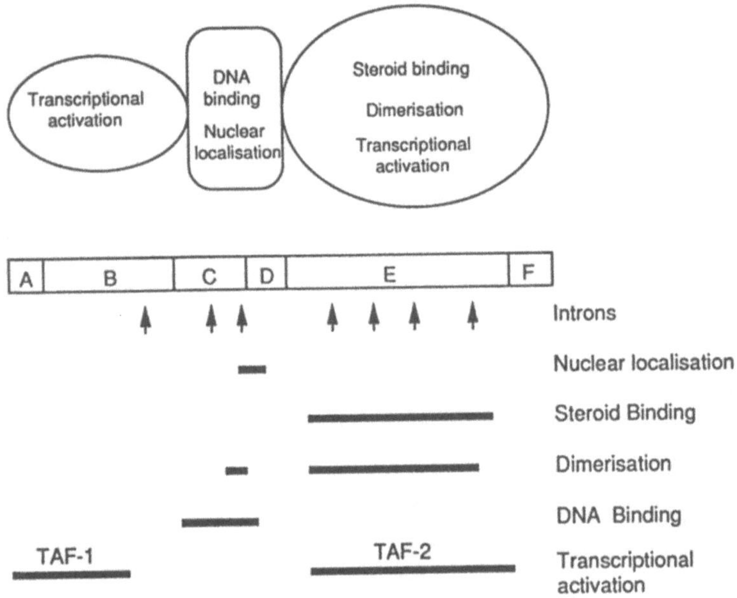

Fig. 1. Structural and functional domains in the oestrogen receptor.
A-F represent regions of the receptor distinguished by their homology with corresponding regions of other receptors [45]. The arrows represent the positions of introns in the gene for the oestrogen receptor.

in oestrogen binding, however, since it can be mutated without affecting the ability of the receptor to bind oestrogen [10]. That it is close to the hormone binding site is supported by examining other mutant mouse receptors which indicated that amino acids between residues 518 and 525 were required for oestrogen binding activity [11].

Interestingly, although mutation of a glycine at position 525 and a methionine and/or serine at positions 521/522 essentially abolished oestrogen binding activity, the mutations did not markedly affect the binding of 4-hydroxytamoxifen to the receptor [11]. The mutant receptors retained the partial agonist activity exhibited by the wild-type receptor in the presence of 4-hydroxytamoxifen. Analysis of the human receptor has shown that mutation of lysines at

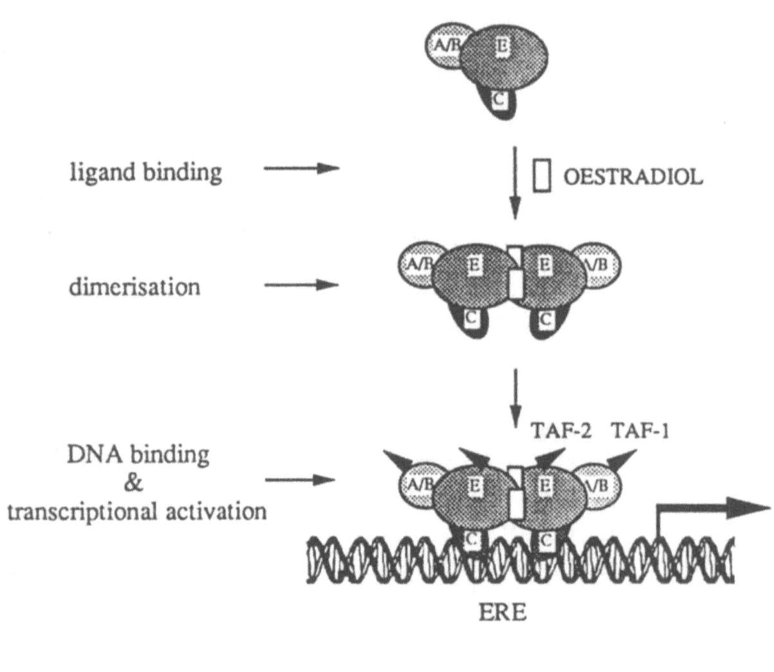

Fig. 2. Model to show the mechanism of action of oestrogen receptors in transcriptional activation.
A-E represent different regions of the receptor (see Fig. 1). ERE is an oestrogen response element and TAF-1/TAF-2 are transcriptional activation functions 1 and 2.

positions 529 and 531 (corresponding to residues 533 and 535, respectively, in the mouse protein) to glutamines reduced its affinity for oestradiol 5 to 10-fold but had no effect on hydroxytamoxifen binding [12]. Thus a number of residues in the C-terminal region of the hormone binding domain are able to confer differential sensitivity to oestrogen and 4-hydroxytamoxifen, suggesting that their binding sites overlap one another but are not completely coincident.

Receptor dimerisation appears to be mediated by two different domains in the protein. The major dimer interface has been mapped in the hormone binding domain but there is also another region in the DNA binding domain which seems to form protein-protein contacts when the receptor is bound to DNA [13]. Some of the residues involved in these interactions have been identified by functional analysis of mutant receptors (Fig. 3). Those in the hormone binding domain have been shown to overlap with residues that are essential for oestrogen binding [10]. It is conceivable, therefore, that the hormone binding pocket is at or near the dimer interface and that hormone binding may result in stabilised dimerisation perhaps on the basis of hydrophobic shielding.

Transcriptional activation by the oestrogen receptor is mediated by at least two distinct activation regions (TAFs): TAF-1 is located in the N-terminal domain while TAF-2 is in the hormone binding domain [14-18]. TAF-1 appears to function constitutively when the receptor is bound to target DNA binding sites whereas TAF-2 depends on oestrogen binding for its transcriptional activity. Their absolute and relative activities vary depending on the cell type and although the types that have been examined are not usually considered target cells for oestrogens it is assumed that differences are likely to mimic the situation in normal target tissues. One type of explanation to account for cell-specific differences is that the activity of different TAFs is regulated by either activators or repressors whose expression or activity is cell dependent.

Molecular Mechanism of Action of Tamoxifen

The main therapeutic antioestrogen that has been used to date is tamoxifen. In fact, as a consequence of metabolism, mainly in the liver, it is converted into 4-hydroxytamoxifen which is approximately 100-fold more potent than tamoxifen itself [19]. Chambon and his colleagues have proposed a model for the action of tamoxifen based on the observation that there are two discrete transcriptional activation regions in the oestrogen receptor, TAF-1 and TAF-2, which are capable of functioning independently [8,17,18]. The activity of TAF-2 is dependent on the binding of hormonal ligand and is negligible in the presence of 4-hydroxytamoxifen whereas the activity of TAF-1 is constitutive once the receptor binds to the target gene. Since 4-hydroxytamoxifen is able to promote the binding of receptor to DNA, it has the potential to stimulate transcription of target genes at least partially (Fig. 4). Therefore, it is likely that tamoxifen would act predominantly as an antagonist on gene promoters on which

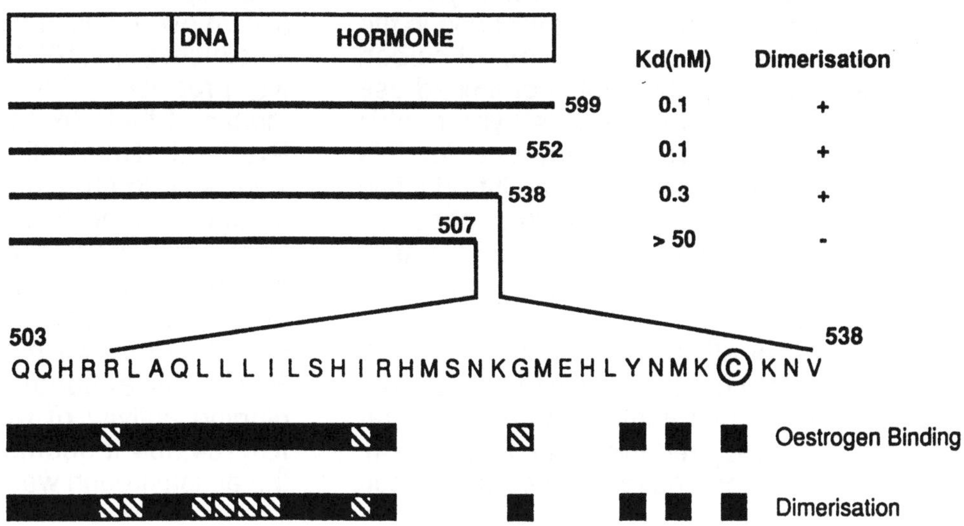

Fig. 3. Residues involved in oestrogen binding and dimerisation overlap, but are not coincident. Striped bars indicate residues which are essential for functional activity and solid bars indicate residues which can be mutated without loss of function. The cysteine residue which is covalently labelled by tamoxifen aziridine and ketononestrol aziridine is marked as C.

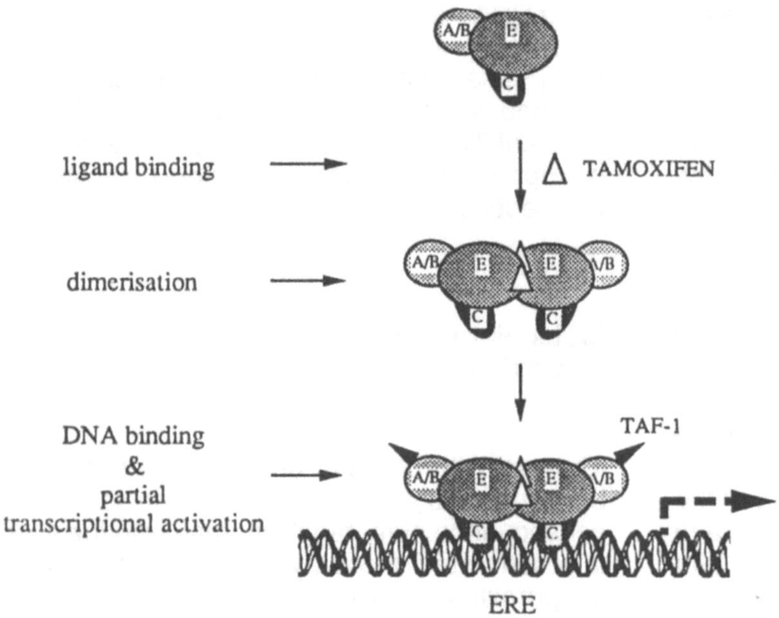

Fig. 4. Model to show the mechanism of action of tamoxifen in transcriptional activation.
For abbreviations see Figure 2.

TAF-2 contributed most activity, but as an agonist when TAF-1 was most active. If both TAF-1 and TAF-2 contributed activity, tamoxifen would act as a mixed agonist/antagonist.

Mechanism of Action of "Pure" Oestrogen Antagonists

The first antioestrogen reported to be devoid of oestrogenic activity was ICI 164,384 [20,21], and as such was referred to as a "pure" antioestrogen. The effectiveness of ICI 164,384 as an antioestrogen depends on an alkylamine side chain at the 7α-position of the B ring in the steroid whose optimum length is 16-18 carbon atoms [22]. ICI 164,384 itself is of limited use as an effective drug because its hydrophobic nature makes for low solubility and for this reason it has been modified by the introduction of fluorine atoms in the side chain to generate ICI 182,780. This antioestrogen also has a higher affinity for the receptor and is therefore more potent [23].

One of the major effects of ICI 164,384 and ICI 182,780 in breast cancer cells is to cause a decrease in the cellular content of oestrogen receptors by markedly reducing their half-life [24]. This effect has been observed not only in cultured cells but also *in vivo,* at least in mouse uterine tissue [25]. The molecular basis for this increased turnover is not completely clear but we have suggested that it might be caused by a disruption in dimerisation in view of some results we obtained in our previous work. We demonstrated that the DNA binding activity of receptors over-expressed in insect or mammalian cells was inhibited by the antioestrogens [26,27] and the ability of analogues of ICI 164,384 with different side-chain lengths to inhibit DNA binding correlated with their ability to inhibit uterine growth *in vivo* [22]. In view of the similarity in the structure of ICI 164,384 and oestradiol we assume that ICI 164,384 binds to similar if not identical sites which we have shown overlap with a region involved in receptor dimerisation [10] (Fig. 3). As a consequence, we proposed that the antioestrogens by means of their 7α side chains sterically interfered with dimerisation and as a consequence were able to reduce the affinity with which the receptor bound to DNA *in vitro* [27,28]. This suggestion was supported by the unusual property of an antibody MP16 which was able to rescue the DNA binding activity of mutant receptors that were defective in dimerisation. Since this antibody also rescued the DNA binding activity of receptors complexed with ICI 164,384 it seems likely that one effect of the antioestrogen was to inhibit dimerisation.

The proposal that ICI 164,384 disrupts dimerisation is controversial because it has been found that the DNA binding activity of the receptor from some sources is not inhibited upon ICI 164,384 binding *in vitro* [27,28]. Moreover, ICI 164,384 binding to the receptor did not prevent DNA binding in transiently transfected cells or when expressed in yeast [18,29]. It has therefore been argued that the antioestrogen must act at a step subsequent to DNA binding [28,29]. One caveat of these particular experiments, however, is that they were performed with chimeric receptors that might exhibit different properties from the wild-type receptor. For example, they may contain additional dimerisation domains that could bypass any effect of "pure" antioestrogens on dimerisation. Since it is apparent that the DNA binding activity of receptors is significantly inhibited only when they are overexpressed [26,27,30], we assume that this gives rise to less stable receptor dimers than normally found in cells. Nevertheless, while it may not normally be possible to dissociate preformed dimers in target cells when they are not overexpressed, it might be possible to prevent the formation of dimers *in vivo* when the receptor is synthesised in the presence of ICI 164,384.

This controversy has been further complicated recently since it has become evident that steroid receptors undergo a process called nucleo-cytoplasmic shuttling. The progesterone and oestrogen receptors have been shown to diffuse from the nucleus into the cytoplasm and, in an energy-dependent process, shuttle back into the cell nucleus so that at equilibrium they appear predominantly nuclear [31]. Immunofluorescence studies showed that the progesterone receptor could associate with and co-translocate a nuclear transport-defective mutant receptor into the nucleus in a progesterone-dependent manner. Corresponding studies with the oestrogen receptor showed that oestrogen and tamoxifen, but not ICI 164,384, promoted the co-translocation [32]. It is likely that co-translocation is mediated by dimerisation through the hormone binding domain. In our own work we have found that, in contrast to oestrogen and tamoxifen, ICI 164,384 and ICI 182780 failed to promote nu-

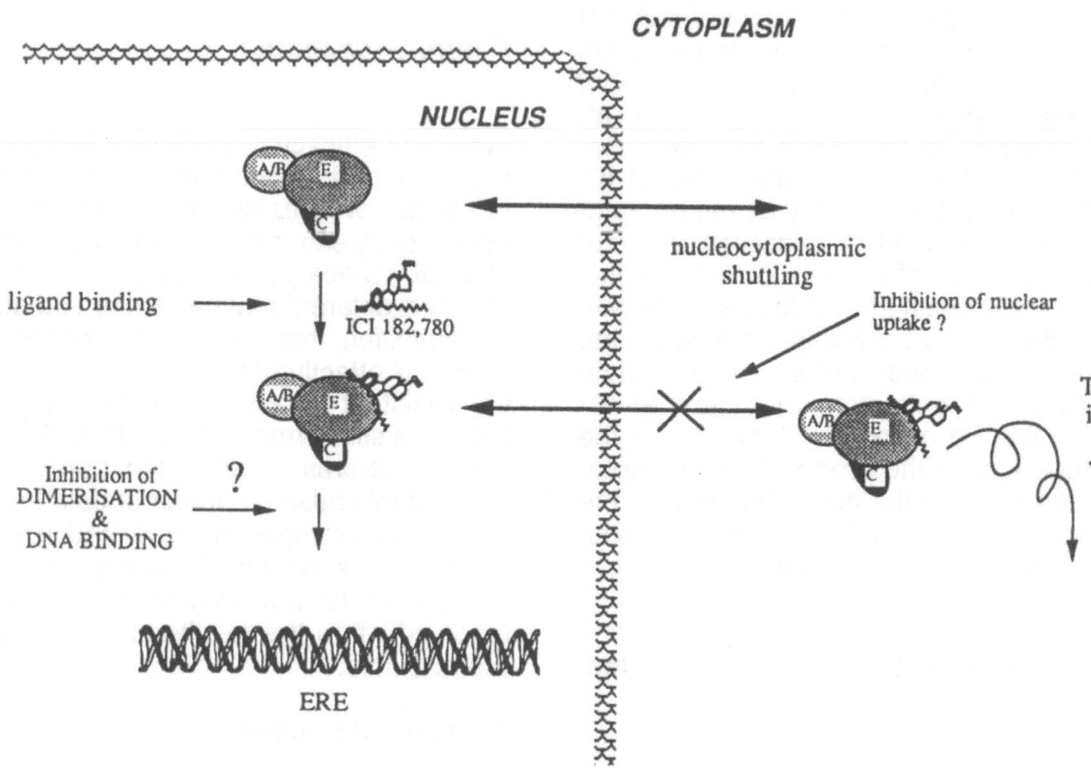

Fig. 5. Model to show the mechanism of action of ICI 182,780 in oestrogen receptor activity. For abbreviations see Figure 2.

clear uptake of the receptor [S. Dauvois, unpublished results]. In view of the potential for these antioestrogens to inhibit dimerisation we favour the suggestion that their inability to promote nuclear uptake might result from impaired dimerisation. In the absence of nuclear uptake it appears that the receptor is more rapidly degraded, perhaps in lysozomes (Fig. 5).

Are ICI 164384 and ICI 182780 Pure Antioestrogens?

Finally, although ICI 164,384 and ICI 182,780 completely inhibit the oestrogen-dependent growth of target cells, they have been found to exhibit some agonistic activity in that they stimulate the expression of progesterone receptors in the uterus [33] and in endometrial carcinoma cell lines [34]. Strictly speaking, therefore, they are not pure antioestrogens but partial agonists. This agonistic activity has been used as an argument against the proposal that ICI 164,384 and ICI 182,780 inhibit receptor dimerisation and DNA binding activity. However, it has yet to be demonstrated that these effects are directly on gene transcription but, assuming that they are, they may not necessarily involve direct binding of the oestrogen receptor to oestrogen response elements. It is conceivable that the effect of ICI 164,384 is not mediated solely by the receptor but might involve another transcription factor such as a member of the Fos or Jun families since they have been shown to associate with several different steroid receptors to stimulate or repress transcription [35-41]. To elucidate the molecular mechanism of action of ICI 164,384 it will be necessary first to map the DNA sequences in the progesterone receptor gene which mediate the agonistic effect of the antioestrogen and then to identify the transcription factors which bind to the element.

What Is the Molecular Basis for Tamoxifen Resistance?

Approximately half the patients whose tumour is oestrogen receptor positive respond to tamoxifen treatment. Unresponsive tumours might arise if the receptor is for some reason insensitive to tamoxifen or simply because the growth of the tumour is completely independent of oestrogen receptor activity. Lack of sensitivity of the receptor to tamoxifen could be due to changes in the receptor or on the other hand might result from metabolism of tamoxifen. Constitutive transcription by the receptor can be generated in model systems by removing the hormone binding domain [17,18]. Such types of variant receptor have been detected in breast cancer samples and therefore offer one potential explanation for tamoxifen insensitivity [42]. Alternatively, alterations in the metabolism of tamoxifen by the tumour itself may result in forms of the drug which lack antagonistic activity or become agonists [43,44]. Even those patients who are successfully treated with tamoxifen often eventually develop drug resistance. This does not usually reflect loss of receptor and is more likely to result from additional changes in the tumour which render it independent of oestrogen receptor activity or alternatively is caused by mutations in the receptor or alterations in the metabolism of tamoxifen as described above.

Future Prospects

While the efficacy of tamoxifen therapy for the treatment of hormone-dependent breast cancer is already well established, clinical trials are now in progress to investigate the action of ICI 182,780. Since ICI 182,780 appears to function by a different mechanism to that described for tamoxifen, there is a strong possibility that it might be effective for the treatment of tamoxifen-resistant breast cancer, providing that the tumour is still hormone dependent. On the other hand, in contrast to tamoxifen, pure antioestrogens might cause a number of deleterious side effects: for example, an increased incidence of osteoporosis would obviously reduce their usefulness. Issues such as these will only be resolved when the results of the clinical trials are available.

Acknowledgements

I should like to thank members of the Molecular Endocrinology Laboratory for lively discussions and for their comments on the manuscript.

REFERENCES

1 Jordan VC: Biochemical pharmacology of antiestrogen action. Pharmacol Rev 1984 (36):245-76

2 Bentley A, Fentiman IS, Rubens RD, Cuzick J, Crossley E, Durrant K, Harris A, Clarke M, Collins R, Godwin J, Gray R, Greaves E, Harwood C, Mead G, Peto R and Wheatley K: Systemic treatment of early breast cancer by hormonal, cytotoxic, or immune therapy: 133 randomised trials involving 31000 recurrences and 24000 deaths among 75000 women. Part 2. Lancet 1992 (339):71-85

3 Love RR, Mazess RB, Tormey DC, Harden HS, Newcomb PA and Jordan VC: Bone mineral density in women with breast cancer treated for at least two years with tamoxifen. Breast Cancer Res Treat 1988 (12):297-302

4 Turken S, Siris E, Seldin E, Seldin D, Flaster E, Hyman G and Lindsay R: Effects of tamoxifen on spinal bone density in women with breast cancer. JNCI 1989 (81):1086-1088

5 Group EBCTC: Effect of adjuvant tamoxifen and cytotoxic therapy on mortality in early breast cancer. N Engl J Med 1988 (319):1681

6 Nayfield SG, Karp JE, Ford LG, Dorr FA and Kramer BS: Potential role of tamoxifen in prevention of breast cancer. JNCI 1991 (83):1450-1459

7 Jensen EV: Overview of the nuclear receptor family. In: Parker MG (ed) Nuclear Hormone Receptors. Academic Press Limited, London 1991 pp 1-13

8 Green S and Chambon P: Nuclear receptors enhance our understanding of transcription regulation. Trends Genet 1988 (4):309-314

9 Harlow KW, Smith DN, Katzenellenbogen JA, Green GL and Katzenellenbogen BS: Identification of cysteine 530 as the covalent attachment site of an affinity-labelling estrogen (ketononestrol aziridine) and antiestrogen (tamoxifen aziridine) in the human estrogen receptor. J Biol Chem 1989 (164):17476-17485

10 Fawell SE, Lees JA, White R and Parker MG: Characterization and colocalization of steroid binding and dimerization activities in the mouse estrogen receptor. Cell 1990 (60):953-962

11 Danielian PS, White R, Hoare SA, Fawell SE and Parker MG: Identification of residues in the estrogen receptor which confer differential sensitivity to estrogen and hydroxytamoxifen. Mol Endocrinol 1992 (7):232-240

12 Pakdel F and Katzenellenbogen BS: Human estrogen receptor mutants with altered estrogen and antiestrogen ligand discrimination. J Biol Chem 1992 (267):3429-3437

13 Kumar V and Chambon P: The estrogen receptor binds tightly to its responsive element as a ligand-induced homodimer. Cell 1988 (55):145-156

14 Danielian PS, White R, Lees JA and Parker MG: Identification of a conserved region required for hormone dependent transcriptional activation by steroid hormone receptors. EMBO J 1992 (11):1025-1033

15 Kumar V, Green S, Stack G, Berry M, Jin JR and Chambon P: Functional domains of the human estrogen receptor. Cell 1987 (51):941-951

16 Lees JA, Fawell SE and Parker MG: Identification of two transactivation domains in the mouse oestrogen receptor. Nucleic Acids Res 1989 (17):5477-5488

17 Tora L, White J, Brou C, Tasset D, Webster N, Scheer E and Chambon P: The human estrogen receptor has two independent nonacidic transcriptional activation functions. Cell 1989 (59): 477-487

18 Webster NJG, Green S, Jin JR and Chambon P: The hormone-binding domains of the estrogen and glucocorticoid receptors contain an inducible transcription activation function. Cell 1988 (54):199-207

19 Jordan VC, Collins MM, Rowsby L and Prestwich G: A monohydroxylated metabolite of tamoxifen with potent antioestrogenic activity. J Endocrinol 1977 (75):305

20 Wakeling AE and Bowler J: Steroidal pure antioestrogens. J Endocrinol 1987 (112):R7-R10

21 Wakeling AE and Bowler J: Biology and mode of action of pure antioestrogens. J Steroid Biochem 1988 (30):141-148

22 Bowler J, Lilley TJ, Pittam JD and Wakeling AE: Novel steroidal pure antiestrogens. Steroids 1989 (54):71-99

23 Wakeling AE, Dukes M and Bowler J: A potent specific pure antiestrogen with clinical potential. Cancer Res 1991 (51):3867-3873

24 Dauvois S, Danielian PS, White R and Parker MG: Antiestrogen ICI 164,384 reduces cellular estrogen receptor content by increasing its turnover. Proc Natl Acad Sci USA 1992 (89):4037-4041

25 Gibson MK, Nemmers LA, Beckman Jr WC, Davis VL, Curtis SW and Korach KS: The mechanism of ICI 164,384 antiestrogenicity involves rapid loss of estrogen receptor in uterine tissue. Endocrinology 1991 (129):2000-2010

26 Fawell SE, White R, Hoare S, Sydenham M, Page M and Parker MG: Inhibition of estrogen receptor-DNA binding by the 'pure' antiestrogen ICI 164,384 appears to be mediated by impaired receptor dimerization. Proc Natl Acad Sci USA 1990 (87):6883-6887

27 Arbuckle ND, Dauvois S and Parker MG: Effects of antioestrogens on the DNA binding activity of oestrogen receptors in vitro. Nucleic Acids Res 1992 (20):3839-3844

28 Sabbah M, Gouilleux F, Sola B, Redeuilh G and Baulieu E-E: Structural differences between the hormone and antihormone estrogen receptor complexes bound to the hormone response element. Proc Natl Acad Sci USA 1991 (88):390-394

29 Pham TA, Elliston JF, Nawaz Z, McDonnell DP, Tsai MJ and O'Malley BW: Antiestrogen can establish nonproductive receptor complexes and alter chromatin structure at target enhancers. Proc Natl Acad Sci USA 1991 (88):3125-9

30 Martinez E and Wahli W: Cooperative binding of estrogen receptor to imperfect estrogen-responsive DNA elements correlates with their synergistic hormone-dependent enhancer activity. EMBO J 1989 (8):3781-3791

31 Guiochon-Mantel A, Lescop P, Christin-Maitre S, Loosfelt H, Perrot-Applanat M and Milgrom E: Nucleocytoplasmic shuttling of the progesterone

receptor. EMBO J 1991 (10):3851-3859
32 Ylikomi T, Bocquel MT, Berry M, Gronemeyer H and Chambon P: Cooperation of proto-signals for nuclear accumulation of estrogen and progesterone receptors. EMBO J 1992 (11):1-14
33 Pasqualini JR, Giambiagi N, Gelly C and Chetrite G: Antiestrogen action in mammary cancer and in fetal cells. J Steroid Biochem Molec Biol 1990 (37):343-348
34 Jamil A, Croxtall JD and White JO: The effect of anti-oestrogens on cell growth and progesterone receptor concentration in human endometrial cancer cells (Ishikawa). J Mol Endocrinol 1991 (6):215-221
35 Gaub M-P, Bellard M, Scheuer I, Chambon P and Sassone-Corsi P: Activation of the ovalbumin gene by the estrogen receptor involves the Fos-Jun complex. Cell 1990 (63):1267-1276
36 Kato S, Tora L, Yamauchi J, Masushige S, Bellard M and Chambon P: A far upstream estrogen response element of the ovalbumin gene contains several half-palindromic 5'-TGACC-3' motifs acting synergistically. Cell 1992 (68): 731-742
37 Diamond MI, Miner JN, Yoshinaga SK and Yamamoto KR: Transcription factor interactions: selectors of positive or negative regulation from a single DNA element. Science 1990 (249): 1266-1272
38 Jonat C, Rahmsdorf HJ, Park KK, Cato ACB, Gebel S, Ponta H and Herrlich P: Antitumor promotion and antiinflammation: down-modulation of AP-1 (Fos/Jun) activity by glucocorticoid hormone. Cell 1990 (62): 1189-1204
39 Schüle R, Rangarajan P, Kliewer S, Ransone LJ, Bolado J, Yang N, Verma IM and Evans RM: Functional antagonism between oncoprotein c-Jun and the glucocorticoid receptor. Cell 1990 (62): 1217-1226
40 Shemshedini L, Knauthe R, Sassone-Corsi P, Pornon A and Gronemeyer H: Cell-specific inhibitory and stimulatory effects of Fos and Jun on transcription activation by nuclear receptors. EMBO J 1991 (10):3839-3849
41 Yang-Yen H-F, Chambard J-C, Sun Y-L, Smeal T, Schmidt TJ, Drouin J and Karin M: Transcriptional interference between c-Jun and the glucocorticoid receptor: mutual inhibition of DNA binding due to direct protein-protein interaction. Cell 1990 (62):1205-1215
42 Fuqua SA, Fitzgerald SD, Chamness GC, Tandon AK, McDonnell DP, Nawaz Z, O'Malley BW and McGuire WL: Variant human breast tumor estrogen receptor with constitutive transcriptional activity. Cancer Res 1991 (51):105-109
43 Osborne CK, Coronado E, Allred DC, Wiebe V and DeGregorio M: Acquired tamoxifen resistance: correlation with reduced breast tumor levels of tamoxifen and isomerization of trans-4-hydroxytamoxifen. JNCI 1991 (83):1477-1482
44 Osborne CK, Wiebe VJ, McGuire WL, Ciocca DR and DeGregorio MW: Tamoxifen and the isomers of 4-hydroxytamoxifen in tamoxifen-resistant tumors from breast cancer patients. J Clin Oncol 1992 (10): 304-310
45 Krust A, Green S, Argos P, Kumar V, Walter P, Bornert JM and Chambon P: The chicken oestrogen receptor sequence: homology with v-erbA and the human oestrogen and glucocorticoid receptors. EMBO J 1986 (5): 891-897

Pure Antioestrogens - A New Horizon in Breast Cancer Therapy?

Alan E. Wakeling

Bioscience I, ZENECA Pharmaceuticals, Alderley Park, Macclesfield, Cheshire SK10 4TG, United Kingdom

The therapeutic value of antioestrogens in breast cancer treatment is well-established. Experience with Nolvadex* (tamoxifen, ICI 46,474) evolved from the first studies in advanced disease more than 20 years ago [1] to application in adjuvant treatment of primary disease [2], and to the initiation of trials of its potential as a chemopreventive agent in women at high risk of developing breast cancer [3,4]. The major advantage of Nolvadex over older alternative, additive or ablative endocrine treatments, is largely a reflection of the ease of oral treatment and the absence of serious side effects. In advanced disease the proportion of patients responding to Nolvadex and the average duration of response are not significantly greater than those obtained with other endocrine treatments. In adjuvant use, Nolvadex achieves benefit in terms both of an extended disease-free interval and survival compared with no treatment [5]. It is also clear that Nolvadex treatment is palliative rather than curative, and that, even amongst patients who respond to treatment, the majority will experience a recurrence of their disease. This clinical experience poses several important questions about future directions for treatment, two of which will be considered here. Firstly, what treatment(s) should be applied in patients relapsing during or after Nolvadex treatment and, secondly, is it possible that a more complete ablation of oestrogen action will provide more effective treatment?

In parallel with the accumulating clinical experience outlined above, understanding of the molecular mode of action of oestradiol and the way in which tamoxifen and other similar antioestrogens affect oestrogen action, provided insight into how more effective oestrogen antagonists might be obtained [6]. Underlying the well-established partial agonist (oestrogenic) activity of tamoxifen, it was shown that the drug competes with oestradiol for binding to oestrogen receptors (ER) but that the tamoxifen-ER complex does not block completely the induction of transcription of oestrogen-responsive genes by oestradiol [7]. The capacity of the tamoxifen-ER complex to signal oestrogen-like effects, in a partially or wholly attenuated manner dependent on the particular cell and gene response measured [6], emphasises the fact that complete ablation of all oestrogen actions cannot be achieved with tamoxifen. Equally, newer treatments designed to reduce the synthesis of oestrogens, for example with aromatase inhibitors, will not achieve complete oestrogen withdrawal. Even complete blockade of oestrogen synthesis from endogenous precursors will not influence the potential action of oestrogens derived from dietary sources [8].

Conceptually, complete blockade of the action of oestrogens in breast cancer patients is a desirable goal which might be achieved by the use of pure antioestrogens. In contrast to partial agonists like tamoxifen, such agents should bind ER with a high affinity without stimulating the transcription of oestrogen-responsive genes. A search for such compounds was initiated in this laboratory and led to the description of ICI 164,384, a 7α-derivative of oestradiol [9] which satisfies the above definition of pure antioestrogens (see [10] for review). A similar, more potent pure antioestrogen, ICI 182,780, has recently been selected for clinical studies [11]. Some of the potential therapeutic advantages of pure versus partial agonist antioestrogens which might emerge, are more

* Nolvadex is a Trade Mark, the property of ZENECA Pharmaceuticals

rapid or complete responses, or a longer-lasting antitumour effect, or both. Experimental evidence whichs supports these assertions is summarised below.

Pure Antioestrogen Treatment in Patients with Advanced Breast Cancer Relapsing During Nolvadex Therapy

Among patients with advanced breast cancer who respond initially to Nolvadex and then relapse on treatment, approximately half benefit from a second course of endocrine therapy, for example with high-dose progestin treatment or an aromatase inhibitor. Thus, it is reasonable to assume that such patients will also respond to pure antioestrogen therapy. However, the key question is whether any additional benefit might accrue with the new agent(s)? Both *in vitro* and *in vivo* studies provide evidence that this may be the case.

Oestrogen-responsive MCF-7 human breast cancer cells grown *in vitro* or as xenografts in nude mice, and long exposed to tamoxifen, overcome the initial inhibitory effect and resume growth [12-15]. *In vitro*, tamoxifen-"resistant" cells remain sensitive to the growth inhibitory action of ICI 164,384 [12]. Thus, tamoxifen-resistant cells are not necessarily cross-resistant to pure antioestrogens. Studies with T47D oestrogen-responsive human breast cancer cells suggest that the mechanism underlying the development of tamoxifen resistance *in vitro* is the outgrowth of subpopulations of cells whose growth is stimulated by tamoxifen, rather than the selective growth of cells which are unaffected by tamoxifen [16]. This mechanism would be consistent with the cells remaining sensitive to ICI 164,384. Also, since pure antioestrogens are devoid of oestrogenic activity, it can be predicted that these agents will not promote the outgrowth of "resistant" cells in the same way as tamoxifen, a prediction that is borne out by our inability to detect any change in the sensitivity of MCF-7 cells after long periods of exposure to ICI 164,384 and the absence of any literature reports describing ICI 164,384-resistant human breast cancer cells.

These observations have very important clinical implications. Clearly, since pure antioestrogens are by definition and characterisation devoid of oestrogenic activity, their therapeutic use will avoid at least one underlying reason for the development of drug resistance. For this reason, it seems reasonable to predict that a longer average duration of response might be sustained than that seen in Nolvadex-treated patients. This prediction is particularly relevant to the choice of first-line endocrine treatment of breast cancer (see following section).

Animal model studies have provided evidence that a similar resistance mechanism might operate *in vivo*. The growth of MCF-7 cells as solid tumours in nude mice is blocked initially by tamoxifen but then resumes [13,14]. That these tumours which develop "resistance" to continued tamoxifen are not resistant in the sense generally understood in cancer therapeutics, was shown in two ways. Re-transplantation studies showed firstly that such tumours would grow only if the host was treated with either tamoxifen or oestradiol and, secondly, that the growth of these tamoxifen-"resistant" tumours is attenuated by the pure antioestrogen ICI 164,384 [17]. The latter observation is consistent with earlier work which showed that pure antioestrogens can block the oestrogenic action of tamoxifen on the uterus or mammary gland [9,11,18], and with the operation, *in vivo*, of a selection pressure like that described *in vitro* [16], which favours the outgrowth of a population of cells dependent on the oestrogenic component of tamoxifen's activity. If this is the case, simple withdrawal of tamoxifen might lead to tumour remission. There is clinical evidence which supports this assertion [19]. However, since tamoxifen can remain in tissues for very long periods after drug withdrawal [20], additive treatment with a pure antioestrogen might further improve response rates.

Although it is not clear what proportion of breast tumours relapse during Nolvadex therapy because they become dependent rather than resistant, there is a sound pharmacological basis for evaluating pure antioestrogen treatment in such patients.

Primary Treatment of Advanced Breast Cancer with Pure Antioestrogen

The key question in this group of patients is whether complete ablation of oestrogen action can be achieved with a pure antioestrogen and, if so, is this likely to lead to improvements in therapeutic response compared with Nolvadex treatment? Evidence from tumour cell and animal studies which predicts a positive answer to these questions will be briefly summarised.

Comparative studies of the growth inhibitory action of tamoxifen and pure antioestrogens on oestrogen-responsive MCF-7 human breast cancer cells *in vitro* revealed that pure antioestrogens are much more potent (approx. 100-fold) [11,21] but, more importantly, are much more effective in reducing the proportion of cells which remain in the actively proliferating fraction [11,21]. This difference was substantial; the proportion of proliferating cells after 5 days of exposure to ICI 182,780 was reduced from 82% in controls to 37% by tamoxifen treatment and to 7% by ICI 182,780 [11]. This difference is attributed to the residual stimulatory (oestrogenic) activity of tamoxifen which, although small, may be amplified by the concurrent presence of serum growth factors [22]. The clear implication of these studies is that pure antioestrogen treatment has the potential to achieve a more complete blockade of oestrogen-stimulated tumour growth than tamoxifen. This may lead to either a more rapid or more complete tumour remission.

A further important distinction between the effects of pure and partial agonist antioestrogens on MCF-7 cells *in vitro* emerged from studies of tumour cell invasiveness. It was shown that both oestradiol and tamoxifen stimulate cell passage through a synthetic basement membrane whereas ICI 164,384 had no effect and also blocked oestrogen-induced invasiveness [23]. ICI 164,384 was also shown to inhibit the capacity of MCF-7 cells to invade cultured chick heart embyro fragments [24]. Thus, pure antioestrogens may be more effective inhibitors of local invasiveness and distant metastasis than tamoxifen.

In studies of the comparative antitumour efficacy of tamoxifen and pure antioestrogens on DMBA-induced rat mammary tumours, it has proved difficult to demonstrate a clear advantage of the pure antagonists [10,25]. It has been argued previously that this may be due to the important role of prolactin in tumour growth since tamoxifen, but not pure antioestrogens, affect prolactin secretion [10]. The complications of this model introduced by differential actions of tamoxifen and pure antioestrogens on the hypothalamus and pituitary gland [25], were avoided in studies in which postmenopausal human breast cancer was more closely modelled by treatment with the LHRH analogue Zoladex* [26]. This treatment effectively castrates the animals and leads to significant tumour involution. Co-administration of ICI 164,384 was shown to accelerate the rate of tumour regression, to increase the proportion of tumours responding and was more effective than Zoladex alone in preventing the appearance of new tumours [26]. In contrast, addition of tamoxifen to Zoladex reduced the apparent efficacy of Zoladex treatment [26]. Thus, total oestrogen ablation achieved with a pure antioestrogen plus Zoladex provided the most effective tumour treatment. Interestingly, the size of the uterus also reflected the differential effects of tamoxifen and ICI 164,384 on cell growth in these studies. The pure antioestrogen reduced further the weight of the uterus compared with Zoladex alone whereas tamoxifen caused an increase [26].

Pure Antioestrogen Treatment in Patients Relapsing on or After Adjuvant Nolvadex Therapy

Treatment choice for patients who relapse during or at some time after adjuvant Nolvadex therapy for primary breast cancer, is a subject of increasing importance because an ever increasing proportion of patients are receiving such treatment. In the absence of any ability to discriminate in individual patients clear, mechanism-based reasons for treatment failure, therapeutic decisions will continue to depend on clinical judgements between the available options. It may be argued that the availability of pure antioestrogens will provide a new treatment option which could reveal novel insights into the causes of treatment failure. Based on the experimental precedents discussed above in the case of recurrence of advanced disease during Nolvadex treatment, there is a sound rationale for treating patients who relapse during adjuvant Nolvadex therapy with pure anti-

* Zoladex is a Trade Mark, the property of ZENECA Pharmaceuticals

oestrogens. The number of patients in this category is likely to increase substantially in the future due to the trend to maintain adjuvant treatment until relapse.

Recent studies on the metabolism of tamoxifen in resistant tumours removed from nude mice indicate that responsive and resistant tumours differ in respect of concentrations of the parent drug and potentially oestrogenic metabolites [27]. Tamoxifen-stimulated tumour growth may be explained by metabolic adaptation of the tumour. Preliminary data indicate that similar changes may occur in patients relapsing on Nolvadex treatment [28,29]. It can be predicted that pure antioestrogens would block the mitogenic effects of oestrogenic tamoxifen metabolites as effectively as they do that of tamoxifen itself. Whether such metabolic adaptations could occur during long-term pure antioestrogen treatment is not known but seems unlikely to occur by the same mechanism(s) because the pure antioestrogens are quite different in structure from tamoxifen.

For patients who relapse at some time after (at least 3 months?) completion of an adjuvant course of Nolvadex, there is no *a priori* reason to exclude a further trial of Nolvadex. However, based again on the arguments deployed above that pure antioestrogens are the more effective inhibitors of tumour cell growth and are less likely to induce treatment failure, it can be argued that a better option is treatment with a pure antioestrogen.

Practical Aspects of Pure Antioestrogen Treatment

In comparative studies of the antioestrogenic potency of ICI 164,384 administered orally or parenterally, it was apparent that the oral bioavailabilty of this agent is poor [9]. Although potency was substantially improved by chemical modification to produce ICI 182,780, oral bioavailability remained poor [11] and necessitated development of an alternative strategy for its therapeutic use. Experimental studies in rats dosed subcutaneously (s.c., or intramuscularly, i.m.) with a variety of oil-based formulations of ICI 182,780, showed that antioestrogenic activity following a single injection could be sustained for long periods. The potential therapeutic utility of such oil-depot formulations was demonstrated by a sustained antitumour action following single s.c. injections in nude mice transplanted with human breast tumours [11]. At the same time, it was necessary to develop short-acting formulations to sustain the high drug exposure essential for toxicological evaluation of ICI 182,780. The latter objective was achieved with a propylene glycol-based formulation and coincidentally provided a formulation suitable for initial clinical pharmacology studies.

In order to predict the likely dose and frequency of treatment in breast cancer patients, the duration of antioestrogenic action of oil depots of ICI 182,780 was measured in monkeys (*Macaca nemestrina*) using magnetic resonance imaging (MRI) of the uterus [30]. Initial studies employed ovariectomised animals where a single i.m. injection of ICI 182,780 was given together with continuous daily injections of oestradiol, and the volume of the endometrium and myometrium was measured weekly by MRI [31]. These studies showed that single injections of ICI 182,780 maintain complete blockade of the uterus in a dose-dependent manner for 3-6 weeks. Repeated injections of 4 mg ICI 182,780/kg at 4-weekly intervals provided increasingly effective blockade of oestrogen-induced uterine proliferation, without significant accumulation of the drug monitored by analysis of plasma drug concentration [30]. The short-acting formulation also effectively blocked oestrogen action completely at a daily dose of 0.1-0.2 mg ICI 182,780/kg. Similarly, when the uterus was maximally stimulated by unopposed oestrogen, treatment with ICI 182,780 caused involution of the uterus at the same rate, and to the same extent as withdrawal of oestrogen, consistent with pure antioestrogenic activity in the primate [30]. These studies set the scene for initial clinical work with ICI 182,780 outlined below.

Several studies following satisfactory completion of the necessary animal toxicology work, as well as an escalating single-dose safety and tolerance study in volunteers, are in progress or scheduled to start shortly. The first two studies were designed to evaluate the clinical pharmacology of the short-acting formulation of ICI 182,780 in two groups of patient volunteers using surrogate endpoints of oestrogen action. The first study in patients undergoing elective hysterectomy for dysfunctional uterine bleeding used ultrasound measurement of the endometrium to assess treatment effects. The second study, in patients with primary breast cancer, employed measurements of tumour oestrogen and progesterone receptor status, the oestrogen-regulated protein pS2, together with Ki67 as an indicator of tumour proliferative capacity. In each study, patients received a daily i.m. injection of ICI 182,780 for 7 days prior to surgery and the measurements described above were made before and after treatment. Both studies are nearing completion but the results remain to be compiled. The drug treatment was well tolerated in all patients.

Further long-term toxicology studies have recently been completed as a prelude to therapeutic studies with the long-acting, oil-depot formulation of ICI 182,780 in patients. The initial trial will be carried out in patients with advanced breast cancer who relapsed during Nolvadex treatment.

Summary

The pharmacology of pure antioestrogens like ICI 182,780 is distinctively different from that of the partial agonist antioestrogens exemplified by tamoxifen. Extensive characterisation of these new agents in oestrogen-responsive cell and animal models of breast cancer provides convincing evidence that pure antioestrogens can block oestrogen action completely. These studies also provide evidence that complete ablation of oestrogen action may lead to one or more of the following advantages in breast cancer therapeutics compared with tamoxifen: tumour responses may be more rapid, more complete or longer-lasting. Clinical trials with ICI 182,780 will reveal whether one or more of these predictions is correct. Finally, model studies have also shown that patients with tumours recurring during tamoxifen therapy may be prime candidates for treatment with ICI 182,780.

REFERENCES

1 Cole MP, Jones CTA and Todd IDH: A new antioestrogenic agent in late breast cancer. An early appraisal of ICI 46,474. Br J Cancer 1971 (25):270-275
2 Smith I: Adjuvant tamoxifen for early breast cancer. Br J Cancer 1987 (57):527-528
3 Poles TJ, Tillyer Cr, Jones AL et al: Prevention of breast cancer with tamoxifen - an update on the Royal Marsden Hospital Pilot Programme. Eur J Cancer Clin Oncol 1990 (26):680-684
4 Nayfield SG, Karp JE, Ford LG et al: Potential role of tamoxifen in prevention of breast cancer. JNCI 1991 (83):1450-1459
5 EBCTCG: Systemic treatment of early breast cancer by hormonal, cytotoxic, or immune therapy. Lancet 1992 (339):1-15
6 Wakeling AE: Pharmacology of antioestrogens. In: Furr BJA and Wakeling AE (eds) Pharmacology and Clinical Uses of Inhibitors of Hormone Secretion and Action. Bailliere Tindall, London 1987 pp 1-19
7 Jordan VC and Murphy CS: Endocrine pharmacology of antiestrogens as antitumor agents. Endoc Rev 1990 (11):578-610
8 Welshons WV, Murphy CS, Koch R et al: Stimulation of breast cancer cells in vitro by the environmental estrogen enterolactone and the phytoestrogenequol. Breast Cancer Res Treat 1987 (10):169-175
9 Wakeling AE and Bowler J: Steroidal pure antioestrogens. J Endoc 1987 (112):R7-R10
10 Wakeling AE: Steroidal pure antiestrogens. In: Lippman ME and Dickson RB (eds) Regulatory Mechanisms in Breast Cancer. Kluwer, Boston 1991 pp 239-257
11 Wakeling AE, Dukes M and Bowler J: A potent specific pure antiestrogen with clinical potential. Cancer Res 1991 (51):3867-3873
12 Lykkesfeldt AE and Sorenson EK: Effect of estrogen and antiestrogens on cell proliferation and synthesis of secreted proteins in the human breast cancer cell line MCF-7 and a tamoxifen resistant variant subline, AL-1. Acta Oncol 1992 (31):131-138
13 Osborne CK, Coronado EB and Robinson JP: Human breast cancer in the athymic nude mouse: cytostatic effects of long-term antiestrogen therapy. Eur J Cancer Clin Oncol 1987 (23):1189-1196
14 Gottardis MM and Jordan VC: Development of tamoxifen-stimulated growth of MCF-7 tumors in athymic mice after long-term antiestrogen administration. Cancer Res 1988 (48):5183-5187
15 Clarke R, Brunner N, Katzenellenbogen BS et al: Progression of human breast cancer cells from hormone-dependent to hormone-independent growth both in vitro and in vivo. Proc Natl Acad Sci USA 1989 (86):3649-3653
16 Graham ML, Smith JA, Jewett PB and Horwitz KB: Heterogeneity of progesterone receptor content and remodeling by tamoxifen characterize subpopulations of cultured human breast cancer cells: analysis by quantitative dual parameter flow cytometry. Cancer Res 1992 (52):593-602
17 Gottardis MM, Jiang S-Y, Jeng M-H and Jordan VC: Inhibition of tamoxifen-stimulated growth of an MCF-7 tumor variant in athymic mice by novel steroidal antiestrogens. Cancer Res 1989 (49):4090-4093
18 Nicholson RI, Gotting KE, Gee J and Walker KJ: Actions of oestrogens and antioestrogens on rat mammary gland development: relevance to breast cancer prevention. J Steroid Biochem 1988 (30):95-103
19 Howell A, Dodwell DJ, Anderson H and Redford J: Response rate after withdrawal of tamoxifen and progestogens in advanced breast cancer. Ann Oncol 1992 (3):611-617
20 Lien EA, Solheim E and Ueland PM: Distribution of tamoxifen and its metabolites in rat and human tissues during steady-state treatment.Cancer Res 1991 (51):4837-4844
21 Musgrove EA, Wakeling AE and Sutherland RL: Points of action of estrogen antagonists and a calmodulin antagonist within the MCF-7 human breast cancer cell cycle. Cancer Res 1989 (49):2398-2404
22 Wakeling AE, Newboult E and Peter SW: Effects of antioestrogens on the proliferation of MCF-7 human breast cancer cells. Mol Cell Endoc 1989 (2):225-234
23 Thompson EW, Katz D, Shima TB et al: ICI 164,384, a pure antagonist of estrogen-stimulated MCF-7 cell proliferation and invasiveness. Cancer Res 1989 (49):6929-6934
24 Bracke ME, Van Larabeke NA, Vyncke BM and Mareel MM: Retinoic acid modulates both invasion and plasma membrane ruffling of MCF-7 human mammary carcinoma cells in vitro. Br J Cancer 1991 (63):867-872
25 Wakeling AE and Bowler J: Biology and mode of action of pure antioestrogens. J Steroid Biochem 1988 (30):141-147
26 Nicholson RI, Walker KJ, Bouzubar N et al: Estrogen deprivation in breast cancer. Ann NY Acad Sci 1990 (595):316-327
27 Osborne CK, Coronado E, Wiebe VJ et al: Acquired tamoxifen resistance correlates with reduced tumor tamoxifen and trans-4-hydroxytamoxifen in human breast cancer. JNCI 1991 (83):1477-1482
28 Osborne CK, Wiebe VJ, McGuire WL et al: Tamoxifen and the isomers of 4-hydroxytamoxifen in tamoxifen-resistant tumors from breast cancer patients. J Clin Oncol 1992 (10):304-310
29 Wiebe VJ, Osborne CK, McGuire WL and DeGregorio MW: Identification of estrogenic tamoxifen metabolite(s) in tamoxifen-resistant human breast tumors. J Clin Oncol 1992 (10):990-994
30 Dukes M, Miller D, Wakeling AE and Waterton JC: Antiuterotrophic effects of a pure antioestrogen, ICI 182,780: magnetic resonance imaging of the uterus in ovariectomized monkeys. J Endocr 1992 (135):239-247
31 Waterton JC, Miller D, Dukes M and Morrell JSW: Oblique NMR imaging of the uterus in macaques: uterine response to estrogen stimulation. Mag Res Med 1991 (20):228-239

Drug Resistance to Antioestrogen Therapy

V. Craig Jordan

Robert H. Lurie Cancer Center, Northwestern University Medical School, 303 East Chicago Avenue, Olsen Pavilion 8250, Chicago, IL 60611, U.S.A.

There are more than 4.5 million women years of experience with the use of tamoxifen (Nolvadex®) for the treatment of breast cancer. During the past two decades, the initial application of tamoxifen as a palliative therapy for the treatment of stage IV breast cancer has now expanded to establish this antioestrogen as the endocrine treatment of choice for all stages of breast cancer. Indeed, the fact that adjunct tamoxifen produces a survival advantage in both node-positive and node-negative breast cancer, and also reduces the incidence of second primary breast cancers by up to 40% [1] has increased enthusiasm to test the worth of tamoxifen to prevent breast cancer in normal women [2].

Tamoxifen has a low incidence of side effects which has resulted in a tendency to maintain patients on tamoxifen therapy for more than 5 years. Tamoxifen also has some positive oestrogen-like effects that maintain bone density [3] and reduces the incidence of fatal myocardial infarction [4]. Tamoxifen maintenance can clearly be an advantage to node-negative breast cancer patients as a hormone replacement therapy but indefinite treatment of stage I and II patients raises the spectre of rapidly progressing disease when drug resistance develops. At present we have no definitive data about the clinical expression of drug resistance to tamoxifen during indefinite therapy because the clinical trials have not been completed as yet. It is therefore appropriate to focus attention on this aspect of the pharmacology of tamoxifen so that suitable strategies can be developed to aid patient care.

This chapter will review the current theories about the mode of action of tamoxifen and then systematically consider the various mechanisms by which a responsive tumour could become either refractory or stimulated by tamoxifen.

Multifaceted Mode of Action of Tamoxifen

Tamoxifen can modulate a variety of systemic, intra and intercellular processes that, in combination, result in the control of tumour growth (Fig. 1 and 2).

Insulin-like growth factor 1 (IGF-1) is known to be a stimulant for breast cancer cell growth *in vitro*, therefore any method that could reduce circulating IGF-1 levels could reduce the growth rate of tumour cells in patients. Tamoxifen causes a significant decrease in circulating IGF-1 levels [5].

Tamoxifen, a non-steroidal antioestrogen, is a competitive inhibitor of oestrogen action at the oestrogen receptor (ER). Adjuvant tamoxifen increases the circulating level of sex hormone binding globulin (SHBG) in postmenopausal women [6], which results in a decrease in the amount of free oestradiol available for competition with tamoxifen at the ER. This would be an indirect mechanism of antioestrogen action.

However, the principal mechanism of action of tamoxifen is focussed on the breast cancer cell and its surrounding stromal environment (Fig. 2). Oestrogens cause an increase in ER-positive cell replication but also a decrease in the synthesis and secretion of transforming growth factor β (TGFβ) that can act as an autocrine (on the same cell) or paracrine (on adjacent cells) growth inhibitor. Tamoxifen not only increases the local production of TGFβ from ER-positive cells but also from adjacent stromal cells [7]. The TGFβ is known to be able to in-

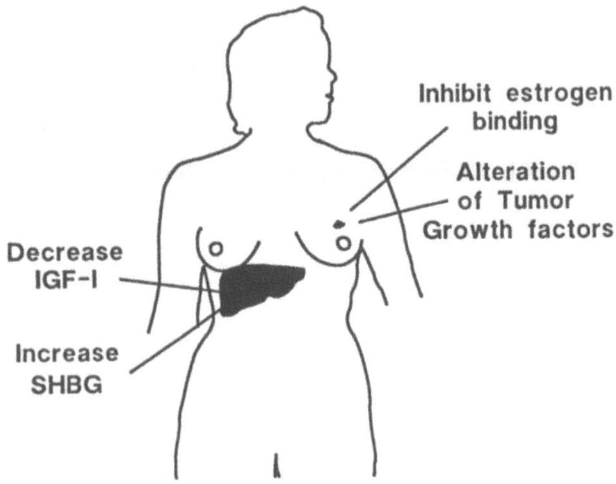

Fig. 1. Multiple mechanisms for the antitumour actions of tamoxifen. IGF1: insulin-like growth factor 1; SHBG: sex hormone binding globulin

hibit cell replications of ER-negative breast cancer cells, an action that could explain why some ER-poor tumours respond to tamoxifen. Indeed the beneficial action of tamoxifen in patients with ER-poor disease [1] suggests that perhaps *all* postmenopausal patients with breast cancer should be given tamoxifen [8]. The beneficial effects in reducing patient mortality far outweigh any detrimental effects caused by iatrogenic disorders or cost considerations.

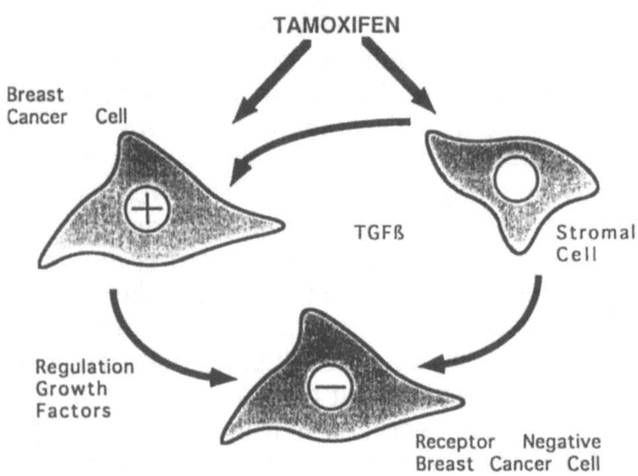

Fig. 2. Potential multicellular mechanism of action of tamoxifen within the breast tumour. TGFß: transforming growth factor ß (an inhibitory paracrine growth factor)

By the end of the century between 4-5 hundred thousand women in the United States could be taking tamoxifen to treat or prevent breast cancer. On a world-wide basis this could be millions of women. It is clearly time to review potential mechanisms of drug failure so that women can be maintained successfully on a longer treatment regimen.

Potential Mechanism of Drug Resistance

The mechanisms to be considered are:
1. Poor absorption or rapid excretion
2. Increasing oestrogen levels
3. Systemic metabolism
4. Local metabolism
5. Loss of oestrogen receptor
6. Mutated oestrogen receptor
7. Altered signal transduction

Poor Absorption or Rapid Excretion

Tamoxifen is readily absorbed following oral administration with peak blood levels occurring within 4 hours. The drug accumulates because there is high (>98%) protein binding and drug levels increase in the plasma until a steady state is achieved. Patients who take 10 mg b.i.d. achieve steady state within 4-6 weeks with a circulating tamoxifen level of 80-150 ng/ml.
Tamoxifen and metabolites are primarily excreted via the bile duct but enterohepatic recirculation occurs to maintain high circulating levels of the drug. The biological half-life of tamoxifen at steady state is 7 days and about 6 weeks is required to reduce circulating levels to zero.
To date, no reports of malabsorption have appeared that would suggest this as a mechanism of drug resistance to tamoxifen.

Increased Oestrogen Levels

The administration of adjuvant tamoxifen to premenopausal women causes an increase in circulating oestrogen levels (oestrone and oestradiol) [9]. Clearly this is of concern for the long-term control of breast cancer with an antioestrogen. High circulating levels of oestradiol could reverse the antitumour action of tamoxifen. Nevertheless, tamoxifen is effective in premenopausal women with stage IV disease, and the drug has antitumour actions as an adjuvant therapy in stage I and stage II disease. There is some evidence [10] that stage IV patients who respond to tamoxifen and subsequently fail can respond to oophorectomy. This suggests that ovarian steroids could have reversed the initial antitumour action of tamoxifen. Laboratory studies *in vivo* have demonstrated that *high* (>2000 pg/ml) circulating levels of oestradiol can reverse the antitumour action of *low* (40 ng/ml) circulating levels of tamoxifen [11]. Clearly, tamoxifen will be more effective in a low oestrogen environment but consistently maintained levels (>100 ng/ml) should prove to be adequate to treat premenopausal women and avoid premature drug failure. Measures to reduce oestrogen levels (oophorectomy or Zoladex®) may prove to be useful as second-line therapy until clinical trials demonstrate the efficacy of simultaneous tamoxifen/Zoladex® therapy to extend tumour responsiveness beyond the response achieved with tamoxifen alone.

Systemic Metabolism

Tamoxifen is converted to a number of well characterised metabolites which are shown in Figure 3. N-Desmethyl tamoxifen is the principal metabolite and circulating levels are usually up to twice those observed for tamoxifen. The biological half-life of N-desmethyltamoxifen is 14 days. Tamoxifen is hydroxylated to form low levels of 4-hydroxytamoxifen, however,

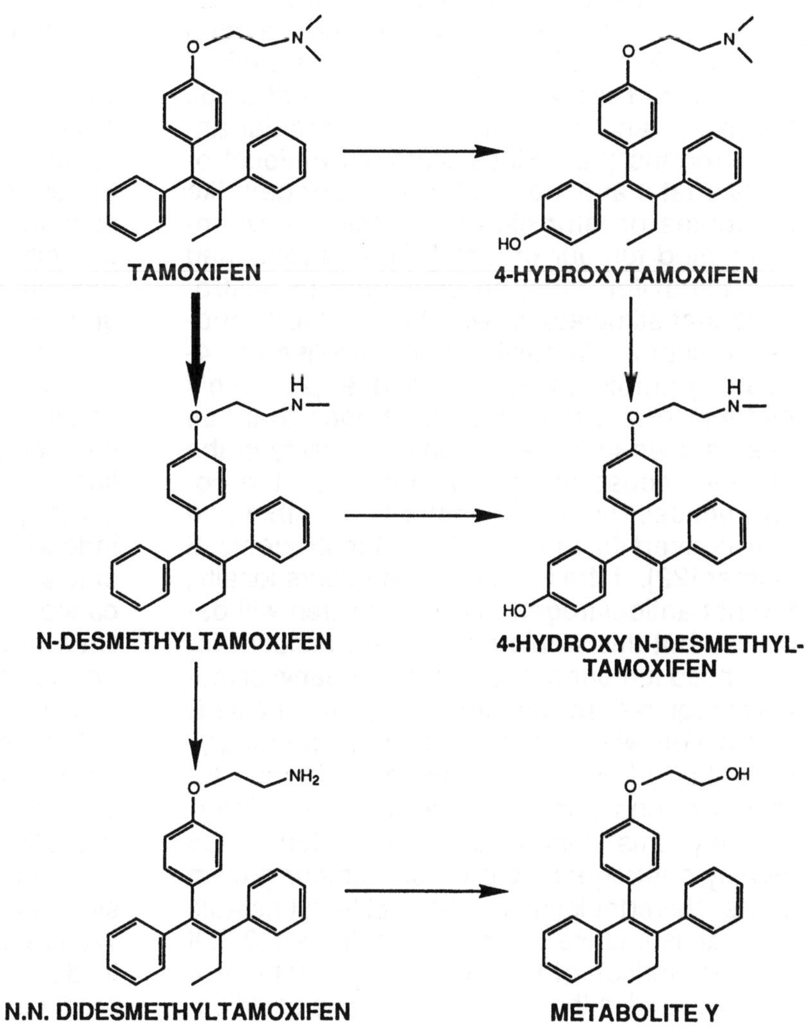

Fig. 3. Metabolites of tamoxifen identified in patient serum. The thickness of the arrows indicates the importance of the metabolic route.

this metabolite has a very high binding affinity for ER [12]. Hydroxylation of N-desmethyltamoxifen occurs in animals and humans to form a minor metabolite with potential antitumour activity [13].

Deamination of N-desmethyltamoxifen to form the weak antioestrogen Metabolite Y has been reported [14]. Although it is possible that the long-term administration of tamoxifen could induce metabolic tolerance and the conversion of tamoxifen to known oestrogens, no biologically significant levels of circulating oestrogenic metabolites have been observed with up to 10 years of tamoxifen treatment [15].

Local Metabolism

It is possible that the tumour cells, or the stromal component, could locally metabolise tamoxifen to potent oestrogens that would stimulate tumour growth. In the laboratory, tamoxifen will stimulate the growth of human breast (MCF-7) or endometrial tumours transplanted into athymic mice [16,17]. The tumours are ER-positive and grow in response to oestradiol, tamoxifen and a variety of non-steroidal antioestrogens [18]. Since steroidal antioestrogens that have none of the oestrogen-like properties of tamoxifen will block tamoxifen-stimulated tumour growth [19], it is reasoned that tamoxifen must be converted to oestrogens that stimulate growth through the oestrogen receptor. Tamoxifen is metabolised to 4-hydroxytamoxifen in the mouse [20]. This metabolite is a potent antioestrogen that has been shown to have antitumour activity in the athymic mouse model [21]. However, the potent antioestrogenic Z isomer is unstable and can convert to the weakly antioestrogenic E isomer [22]. If the isomerisation occurs locally, the net antioestrogenicity of tamoxifen will decrease but this would not, *per se*, account for increased tumour growth; an oestrogenic stimulus is required. Minute amounts of metabolite E (tamoxifen without the dimethyl amino-ethane side chain) have been detected in human tumours during tamoxifen therapy [23]. Unfortunately, this metabolite of tamoxifen is too weakly oestrogenic to promote tumour growth alone. Nevertheless, the metabolite is unstable and can isomerise to a potent oestrogen [22]. If large quantities of this oestrogenic metabolite accumulated in the tumours, then this could account for tamoxifen-stimulated tumour growth by competing out antioestrogenic ligands at the ER. This hypothesis [24] is summarised in Figure 4. We have recently addressed the question of metabolite isomerisation as the mechanism of tamoxifen-stimulated growth by determining the ability of tamoxifen derivatives, which cannot isomerise, to cause tumour growth. Since we have found that tumour growth is adequately supported by non-isomerisable derivatives of tamoxifen, it is unlikely that local metabolite instability is responsible for tamoxifen-stimulated growth. It is perhaps more likely that clones of cells that are extremely sensitive to the intrinsic activity of tamoxifen as an oestrogen are selected and gain a dominant growth advantage. Needless to say, the mechanism of signal transduction that converts an antagonist to an agonist is an area of great current interest within the molecular biology community.

Loss of the Oestrogen Receptor

Oestrogen responsiveness of tissues and tumours is correlated with the presence or absence of the ER. Breast cancer requires oestrogen to promote the process of carcinogenesis and it is generally accepted that tumours are initially ER positive but eventually lose the receptor and become hormone independent for growth.

It is an important current goal of laboratory research to develop models of human breast cancer progression. The objective is to study the biological processes involved in the evolution of hormone dependency in order to find a strategy to prevent, or at least delay, hormone-independent growth. Regrettably, there are only a few hormone-dependent human breast cancer cell lines. Both ZR-75 and MCF-7 cell lines have been used to develop antioestrogen-resistant or oestrogen-independent sublines but invariably the tumour cells retain the ER. In contrast, T47D breast cancer cells, which are ER-positive and oestrogen-responsive for growth, do lose the ER if the cells are maintained in an oestrogen-free environment for many months [25]. The cloned cells are insensitive to both oestrogens and antioestrogens. We are currently using this new model system to devise ways to reactivate the ER gene to produce functional receptor.

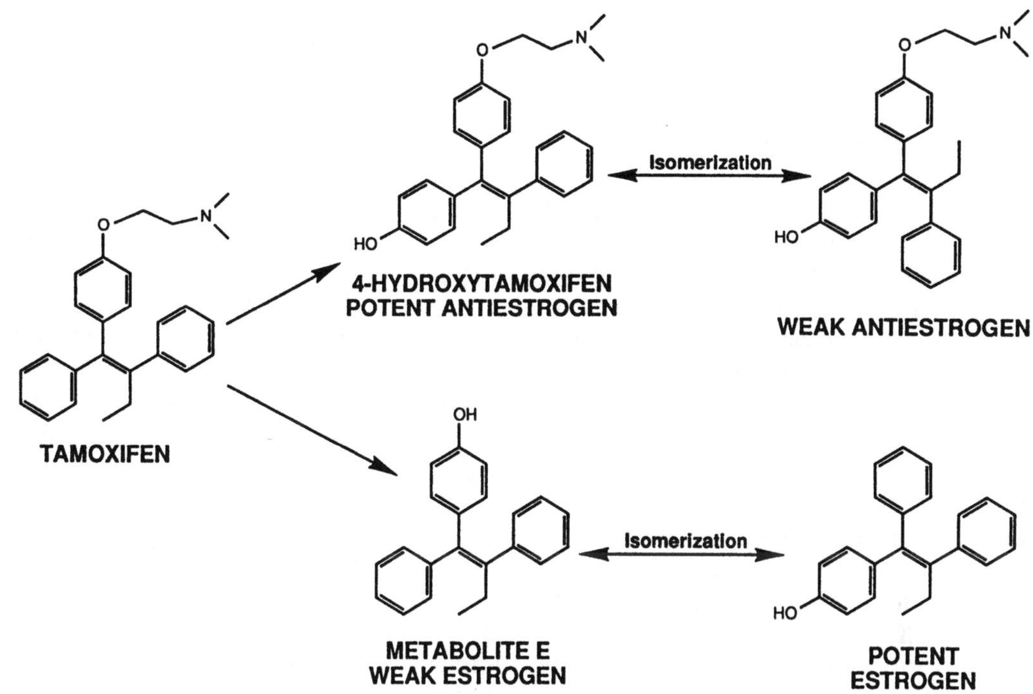

Fig. 4. Potential metabolites of tamoxifen within tamoxifen-stimulated MCF-7 breast tumours, their stability and pharmacological properties

ER genes have been transfected into receptor-negative animal and human cell lines with varying degrees of success [26,27]. High levels of receptor results in a cidal effect from oestrogen treatment [28]. In related experiments we have transfected the ER gene into the ER-negative breast cancer cell line MDA-MB-231 [29]. We chose to develop cell lines that contain levels comparable to those observed in hormone-responsive cells, i.e., approximately 150-300 fmol/mg cytosol protein. Oestradiol decreases the growth rate of transfected breast cancer cells, an effect that is blocked by pure antioestrogens. It is possible that the selective re-activation or transfection of cancer cells with steroid receptor could prove to be a novel therapeutic strategy to control previously refractory disease.

Mutated Oestrogen Receptor

There is much interest in determining the biological relevance of mutated steroid hormone receptors. Laboratory models have demonstrated that specific mutations of the androgen [30] and progesterone receptor [31] can change the pharmacology of antiandrogens and antiprogestins to full agonist molecules. It is therefore possible that mutations in the ER could change the pharmacology from antioestrogens to oestrogens and explain tamoxifen-stimulated growth in tumours. Screening of clinical tumour material has resulted in the identification of several mutations of the ER [32], but the biological relevance of the findings is unclear. However, it is possible to examine the impact of point mutations of the ER on the pharmacology of antioestrogens under laboratory conditions. If MDA-MB-231 cells are transfected with either a wild type ER gene or an ER gene with a gly-to-val mutation at amino acid 400, the resulting transfectants will respond to oestrogen by decreasing growth rate [29]. This then becomes a laboratory model to determine the degree of oestrogenicity expressed by a test molecule under controlled conditions. Pure antioestrogens prevent the inhibitory effect of oestradiol in both wild-type and mutant transfectants [29]. In contrast, the antioestrogens 4-hydroxytamoxifen [33] and RU39411 [34], which are partial oestrogens with antioestrogenic properties in the wild-type transfectants, only express oestrogenic activity in the mutant transfectants. Clearly these data indicate that the pharmacology of antioestrogen can be changed to express fully oestrogenic properties. Should mutations of the ER be found in clinical specimens that are suspected of playing a role in the drug resistance to tamoxifen, the cDNA could be transfected into receptor-negative cells in the laboratory to confirm the suggestion as a fact.

Altered Signal Transduction

It is possible that hormone-independent cells could still synthesise a normal ER but either the local environment or additional subcellular factors have changed. This would prevent the hormone (or antihormone) receptor complex either from binding with other transcription factors or the complex binding adequately to oestrogen response elements (EREs).

The local environment of growth factors can alter hormone and antihormone responsiveness. Epidermal growth factor can stimulate cell replication and can potentially reverse the inhibitory effects of antioestrogen on oestrogen-stimulated growth [35,36]. Indeed, the increased local concentration of growth factors within a heterogeneous tumour may be the reason why some ER-positive tumours (that are PR negative) do not respond to tamoxifen or other antihormonal therapy [37].

Alternatively the receptor may no longer respond to either oestrogens or antioestrogens. Early studies with drug resistance to the antioestrogen LY117018 demonstrated that an ER-positive clone of MCF-7 cells could continue to grow in an antioestrogenic environment [38]. The receptor was shown to have the same sequence as the wild-type hormone-responsive MCF-7 cell line [39]. Similarly we have described [40] an ER-positive clone of MCF-7 cells that does not respond to either oestrogens or antioestrogens for growth. Oestradiol does not stimulate PR production but the ER sequence is not mutated. Clearly there is a fundamental alteration in the signal transduction mechanism that controls replication but a vestigial receptor still remains. An intervention that could resolve the aberrant control mechanism might potentially become a valuable new treatment strategy.

Summary and Conclusions

The ubiquitous use of tamoxifen for the treatment of breast cancer has not only provided the clinical community with a safe and effective therapy, it has also provided an insight into the molecular mechanisms of hormone-dependent growth.

A fundamental piece of information is missing from our knowledge that might be obtained by the research strategies currently being investigated in the laboratory. We are ignorant about the precise and specific control mechanisms that regulate the activation of the ER gene. The current experiments on the drift of hormone-dependent to independent growth through the controlled loss of the ER are an important start to find critical steps in the biochemistry that might respond to therapeutic modulation. Obviously it must be a goal of laboratory research to elucidate the cascade of events that subverts effective transcriptional control through ER. Conversely, it may be equally productive to discover precise ways to maintain receptor control. Cell-specific receptor reactivation could become a powerful tool for the molecular biologist to apply to therapeutic research. The clues obtained from understanding receptor mechanisms in breast cancer could become an important first step in developing strategies to treat all cancers.

REFERENCES

1 Early Breast Cancer Trialists Collaborative Group: Systemic treatment of early breast cancer by hormonal, cytotoxic or immune therapy. Lancet 1992 (i):1-15, 71-85

2 Fisher B: The evolution of paradigms for the management of breast cancer: A personal perspective. Cancer Res 1992 (52):2371-2383

3 Love RR, Mazess RB, Borden HS, Epstein S, Newcomb PA, Jordan VC, Carbone PP and DeMets DL: Effects of tamoxifen bone mineral density in postmenopausal women with breast cancer. N Engl J Med 1992 (326):852-856

4 MacDonald CC and Stewart HJ: Fatal myocardial infarction in the Scottish adjuvant tamoxifen trial. Br Med J 1991 (303):435-437

5 Pollak M, Costantino J and Polychronakos C: Effect of serum insulin-like growth factor 1 levels in stage I breast cancer patients. JNCI 1990 (82):1693-1697

6 Jordan VC, Fritz NF and Tormey DC: Long-term adjuvant therapy with tamoxifen: Effects on sex hormone binding globulin and antithrombin III. Cancer Res 1987 (47):4577-4579

7 Butta A, MacLennan K, Flanders KC, Sacks NPM, Smith I, McKinna A, Dowsett M, Wakefield LM, Sporn MB, Baum M and Coletta AA: Induction of transforming growth factor ß1 in human breast cancer *in vivo* following tamoxifen treatment. Cancer Res 1992 (52):4261-4264

8 Jordan VC: Should all postmenopausal women with a diagnosis of breast cancer receive tamoxifen? Postgrad Gen Surg (in press)

9 Jordan VC, Fritz NF, Langan Fahey S, Thompson M and Tormey DC: Alteration of endocrine parameters in premenopausal women with breast cancer during long-term adjuvant tamoxifen monotherapy. JNCI 1991 (83):1488-1491

10 Sawka CA, Pritchard KI, Paterson DJA, Thomsen DB, Shelley WE, Meyers RE, Mobbs BC, Mulkin A and Meakin JW: Role and mechanism of action of tamoxifen in premenopausal women with metastatic breast cancer. Cancer Res 1986 (46):3152-3156

11 Iino Y, Wolf DM, Langan Fahey SM, Ricchio ME, Johnson DA and Jordan VC: Reversible control of oestradiol-stimulated growth of MCF-7 tumours by tamoxifen in the athymic mouse. Br J Cancer 1991 (64):1019-1024

12 Jordan VC, Collins MM, Rowsby L and Prestwich G: A monohydroxylated metabolite of tamoxifen with potent antiestrogenic activity. J Endocrinol 1977 (73):305-316

13 Lien EH, Solheim E, Kuinnsland S and Veland PM: Identification of 4-hydroxy-N-desmethyltamoxifen as a metabolite of tamoxifen in human bile. Cancer Res 1988 (48):2304-2308

14 Jordan VC, Bain RR, Brown RR, Gosden B and Santos MA: Determination and pharmacology of a new hyroxylated metabolite of tamoxifen observed in patient sera during therapy for advanced breast cancer. Cancer Res 1983 (43):1446-1450

15 Langan Fahey SM, Tormey DC and Jordan VC: Tamoxifen metabolites in patients on long-term adjuvant therapy for breast cancer. Eur J Cancer 1990 (26):883-888

16 Gottardis MM and Jordan VC: Development of tamoxifen-stimulated growth on MCF-7 tumors in athymic mice after long-term antiestrogen administration. Cancer Res 1988 (48):6183-5187

17 Satyaswaroop PG, Zaino RJ and Mortel R: Estrogen-like effects of tamoxifen on human endometrial carcinoma transplanted into nude mice. Cancer Res 1984 (44):4006-4010

18 Gottardis MM, Ricchio ME, Satyaswaroop PG and Jordan VC: Effect of steroidal and nonsteroidal antiestrogens on the growth of a tamoxifen stimulated human endometrial carcinoma (EnCa101) in athymic mice. Cancer Res 1990 (50):3189-3192

19 Gottardis MM, Jiang SY, Jeng MH and Jordan VC: Inhibition of tamoxifen stimulated growth of an MCF-7 variant in athymic mice by novel steroidal antiestrogens. Cancer Res 1989 (49):4090-4093

20 Robinson SP, Langan Fahey SM, Johnson DA and Jordan VC: Metabolites, pharmacodynamics and pharmacokinetics of tamoxifen in rats and mice compared to the breast cancer patient. Drug Metab and Disp 1991 (19):36-43

21 Gottardis MM, Robinson SP and Jordan VC: Estradiol stimulated growth of MCF-7 tumors implanted in athymic mice: A model to study the tumoristatic action of tamoxifen. J Steroid Biochem 1988 (20):311-314

22 Murphy CS, Langan-Fahey SM, McCague R and Jordan VC: Structure-function relationships of hydroxylated metabolites of tamoxifen that control the proliferation of estrogen responsive T47D breast cancer cells *in vitro*. Mol Pharmacol 1990 (38):737-743

23 Wiebe VJ, Osborne CK, McGuire WL and DeGregario M: Identification of estrogenic tamoxifen metabolite(s) in tamoxifen-resistant human breast tumors. J Clin Oncol 1992 (10)990-994

24 Osborne CK, Coronado E, Allred DC, Wiebe V and DeGregorio M: Acquired tamoxifen (TAM) resistance: Correlation with reduced breast tumor levels of tamoxifen and isomerization of trans-4-hydroxytamoxifen. JNCI 1991 (83):1477-1480

25 Murphy CS, Pink JJ and Jordan VC: Characterization of a receptor-negative, hormone non-responsive clone derived from T47D human breast cancer cell line kept under estrogen free conditions. Cancer Res 1990 (50):7285-7292

26 Watts CK, Parker MG and King RJ: Stable transfection of the oestrogen receptor gene into a human osteosarcoma cell line. J Steroid Biochem 1989 (34):483-490

27 Touitou I, Mathieu M and Rochefort H: Stable transfection of the estrogen receptor cDNA into HELA cells induces estrogen responsiveness of endogenous cathepsin D-gene but not of growth. Biochem Biophys Res Coman 1990 (169):109-115

28 Kushner PJ, Hart E, Shine J, Greene GL and Baxter J: Construction of cell lines that express high levels of the human estrogen receptor and are killed by estrogens. Mol Endocrinol 1990 (4):1465-1473

29 Jiang SY and Jordan VC: Growth regulation of estrogen receptor negative breast cancer cells

transfected with cDNAs for estrogen receptor. JNCI 1992 (84):580-591
30 Schurrmans ALG, Bolt J, Veldscholte J and Mulder E: Stimulator effects of antiandrogens on LNCaP human prostate tumor cell growth EGF receptor level and acid phosphatase secretion. J Steroid Biochem Mol Biol 1990 (37):849-853
31 Vegeto E, Allan GF, Schrader WT, Tsai MJ, McDonnell DP and O'Malley BW: The mechanism of RU486 antagonism is dependent on the conformation of the carboxyterminal tail of the human progesterone receptor. Cell 1992 (69):703-713
32 Murphy LC: Estrogen receptor variants in human breast cancer. Mol Cell Endocrinol 1990 (74):C83-C86
33 Jiang SY, Langan-Fahey SM, Stella A, McCague R and Jordan VC: Point mutation of the estrogen receptor (ER) in the ligand binding domain changes the pharmacology of antiestrogens in ER-negative breast cancer cells stably expressing cDNAs for ER. Mol Endo 1992 (6):2167-2174
34 Jiang SY, Parker CJ and Jordan VC: A model to describe how a point mutation of the estrogen receptor alters the structure function relationship of antiestrogens. Breast Cancer Res Treat (in press)
35 Konga M and Sutherland RL: Epidermal growth factor partially reverses the inhibitory effects of antiestrogens on T47D human breast cancer growth. Biochem Biophys Res Comm 1987 (146):739-745
36 Cormier EM and Jordan VC: Contrasting ability of antiestrogens to inhibit MCF-7 growth stimulated by estradiol or epidermal growth factor. Eur J Cancer Clin Oncol 1989 (25):57-63
37 Cormier EM, Wolf MF and Jordan VC: Decrease in estradiol stimulated progesterone receptor production in MCF-7 cells by epidermal growth factor and possible clinical implications for paracrine regulated breast cancer growth. Cancer Res 1989 (49):576-580
38 Brozert DA, Greene GL, Lippman ME: Selection and characterization of a breast cancer cell line resistant to the antiestrogen LY117018. Endocrinology 1985 (117):1409-1415
39 Mallick A and Chambon P: Characterization of the estrogen receptor in two antiestrogen resistant cell lines LY2 and T47D. Cancer Res 1990 (50):333-338
40 Jiang SY, Wolf DM, Yingling JM, Chang C and Jordan VC: An estrogen receptor positive MCF-7 clone that is resistant to antiestrogens and estradiol. Mol Cell Endocrinol 1992 (90):77-86

Antiprogestational Treatment of Breast Cancer: Preclinical and Clinical Experience with Different Antiprogestins

J.G.M. Klijn, B. Setyono-Han, H.J. Sander and J.A. Foekens

Division of Endocrine Oncology, Rotterdam Cancer Institute/Dr. Daniel den Hoed Cancer Centre, Groene Hilledijk 301, 3075 EA Rotterdam, The Netherlands

Many steroid and peptide hormones, growth factors and other trophic substances are involved in the growth regulation of breast cancer [1,2]. Endocrine treatment of breast cancer is designed to decrease plasma concentrations of one or more of these hormones and growth factors or to antagonise the biological effects of these trophic substances directly at the level of the tumour cells. The involvement of so many hormones and other factors offers many points of action for endocrine therapy, both directly and indirectly. Endocrine therapy of breast cancer consists in a variety of both medical and surgical ablative treatment modalities, but ablative therapy is increasingly replaced by medical treatment such as antioestrogens, high-dose progestins, androgens, aromatase inhibitors, luteinising hormone-releasing hormone analogues (LHRH-A), somatostatin analogues and prolactin inhibitors [2]. Oestrogens have fallen into disuse because antioestrogen treatment with tamoxifen showed much less side effects than treatment with high-dose oestrogens. High-dose progestins still form an important endocrine treatment modality, especially as second-line treatment after tamoxifen, but due to their glucocorticoid properties cause a number of undesirable side effects such as body weight gain and Cushingoid symptoms.

Antiprogestins form a new category of antihormonal agents of potential interest in the treatment of cancer, especially for progesterone receptor (PgR) containing tumours. Initially, the first antiprogestational agent mifepristone (RU38486) [3] was used [4-17], but recently several other antiprogestins have become available for experimental and clinical application [8,14,18-23]. In the mid 1980s Rochefort and coworkers [4-6] demonstrated growth inhibitory effects of mifepristone on human breast cancer cells *in vitro*. Their results stimulated us to apply this drug *in vivo*, both in experimental mammary tumour models [9-15,18] and in a clinical trial [12]. Table 1 summarises the differences in effects between progestins and antiprogestins observed *in vitro* and *in vivo* as reported in the initial publications [4-6,9-13]. In this paper we will review the results of our studies on antiprogestins performed during the last 7 years. For an extensive recent review on (anti)progestins and breast cancer we refer to the excellent paper of Horwitz [8].

In Vitro Studies on Human Breast Cancer Cell Lines

The human breast cancer cell lines MCF-7, MDA-MB-231, T-47D, Evsa-T and ZR-75.1 were maintained in continuous culture in their respective complete growth media [24]. As experimental media we used serum-free medium (SFM), steroid-depleted serum-containing medium (DCC-medium) or complete medium with or without the addition of hormones and/or antihormones. Viable cell numbers were measured by the colorimetric MTT assay and the cell cycle distribution of the tumour cells by dual parameter flow cytometry as described previously [25]. The following test substances were used: oestradiol (oestrogen), tamoxifen-citrate and hydroxytamoxifen (antioestrogens), ORG 2058 (progestin), RU 38486 and ORG 31710 (antiprogestins).

In an initial experiment MCF-7 cells were cultured during 7 days in medium supplemented with 10% DCC human male serum with or without oestradiol ($8x10^{-11}$M), tamoxifen ($4 x10^{-8}$ M) or mifepristone ($3.6x10^{-8}$M). No effect of mifepristone was found on the growth of unstimulated MCF-7 cells. However, mifepristone fully abolished ($p<0.005$) the oestradiol-stimulated growth just like tamoxifen [10].
In a further series of 4 experiments culturing MCF-7 cells in SFM there was a dose-dependent increase in the percentage of cells in S-phase after incubation for 24 hours with mifepristone (9-31% by 1-100 nM, 50-56% by 1-10 μM) compared to control cultures (5-16%). Also oestradiol (60% in S-phase) and ORG 2058 stimulated cells to switch to the S-phase, but the stimulatory effect of ORG 2058 (39-66% cells in S-phase) was partly counteracted by 10 μM mifepristone (30-45% in S-phase after administration of both agents) [15]. During long-term incubations of 7 days in SFM, single treatment with mifepristone showed again a dose-dependent stimulatory effect with a clear increase in the number of cells treated with 1 μM. This concentration did not block the growth stimulatory effect of ORG 2058 [15].
Recently we tested the effects of the progestin ORG 2058 and the antiprogestins mifepristone and ORG 31710 on the 5 breast cancer cell lines. Again the highest concentrations (10^{-6}M) of the antiprogestins caused a significant prolonged stimulation of MCF-7 cell proliferation, up to 4.6-fold with mifepristone and 4.0-fold with ORG 31710 by day 9, suggestive of the presence of progesterone agonistic effects. Under the serum-free conditions used, the proliferation of none of the other cell lines tested, i.e., MDA-MB-231 (ER^-/PgR^-), T-47D ($ER^{\pm}/PgR^{++}$), and ZR-75.1 (ER^+/PgR^+) cells, was affected by the antiprogestins.
In DCC-medium, both antiprogestins inhibited the oestrogen-stimulated proliferation of the PgR-rich T-47D cells in a dose-dependent way, as determined on day 7. Inhibition of cell proliferation by the antiprogestins was not observed in the absence of oestradiol. On the other hand, in complete growth medium both antiprogestins stimulated proliferation of T-47D cells, up to 80% for ORG 31710 and up to 100% for mifepristone, as determined after 10 days of culture. The proliferation of the other cell lines in complete growth medium was not or marginally affected by either antiprogestin.
Therefore, it can be concluded that antiprogestins can both stimulate and inhibit breast cancer cell growth *in vitro*, dependent on type of cell line, culture medium and concentration of the drug used.

In Vivo Effects in Rats with DMBA-Induced Mammary Tumours

Effects of Treatments on Tumour Growth

Prophylactic treatment

Prophylactic treatment with mifepristone (10 mg/kg/day) for 3 weeks starting from the day of the first DMBA injection resulted in a doubling of the average tumour latency period [10]. The first appearance of the mammary tumours was shown after 39 days in the control group vs 81 days in the treated group ($p<0.005$).

Antitumour effects in rats with palpable tumours

In initial experiments we tested the efficacy of subcutaneous treatment with mifepristone [9-11,13]. Tumour growth was inhibited by 75-90% compared to controls without significant differences between the doses used (2.5, 10 and 40 mg/kg/day). Treatment with mifepristone appeared more effective ($p<0.01$) than treatment with high dosages (2.5 and 10 mg/kg/day) of the progestin megestrol acetate (40% tumour growth inhibition) and slightly more effective than tamoxifen (0.4 mg/kg/day), i.e., 75% inhibition of tumour growth (Fig.1).
Later on we compared the antitumour efficacy of 2 new antiprogestins (ORG 31710 and ORG 31806) with that of mifepristone by oral treatment [14,18]. It was found that these new compounds were slightly more effective than mifepristone, resulting even in a tumour regression of approximately 20% with ORG 31710 (5 mg/kg/day) when the total initial tumour area was ≥ 500 mm^2 before the start of treatment. Using 4 different dosages of ORG 31710 (0.8, 2, 5 and 10 mg/kg/day), a clear dose-dependent antitumour effect was observed.
Most interesting were the results of combined treatment modalities. Combined antiprogestational antioestrogenic treatment with mifepris-

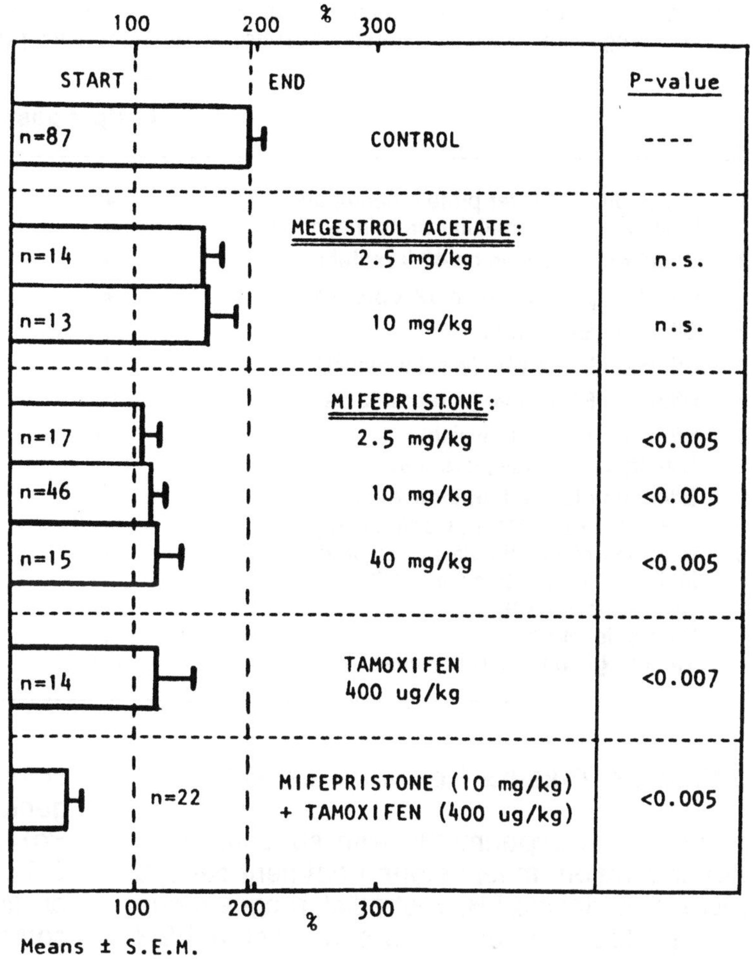

Fig 1. Relative effects on mammary tumour load after different treatments for 3 weeks (from ref. 14). Results are means ± SEM. The number of animals is indicated in the bars. P-value denotes the statistical significance vs control. Initial tumour load = 100%. n.s. = not significant.

tone and tamoxifen (Fig. 1) led to a clear additive antitumour effect resulting in 50% tumour regression [13], while the combination of ORG 31710 and tamoxifen was even more effective (64% tumour regression) [18]. These results are at least as good as those obtained by surgical castration or medical castration by daily buserelin injections (50% tumour regression). The best antitumour effects were observed after treatment with the combination of LHRH-agonist implants (buserelin or goserelin) and an antiprogestin, i.e., 75% tumour regression [13].

Effects on Organ Weight

In the initial experiments where mifepristone was administered subcutaneously, increased weights of the pituitary, ovaries and uterus were found without a change in adrenal weight [9-11,13]. On histological examination the ovaries showed large cystic follicles and unruptured corpora lutea [11]. In normal rats mifepristone caused persistent vaginal cornification, ballooning of the uterus and a dissociation between ovulation and luteolysis in the presence of high plasma oestradiol and progesterone levels [11]. These biological effects can be explained by unopposed oestrogen activity due to blockade of the progesterone receptor. In further experiments where the three antiprogestins were given orally no significant changes in ovarian weight were found.

Treatment with high-dose progestin, megestrol acetate, induced the opposite effects (Table 1), i.e., a decrease in the weight of all organs (pituitary, ovaries, uterus and adrenals). Treatment with tamoxifen or LHRH agonists with or without an antiprogestin caused a decrease in the weight of the ovaries and uterus, while treatment with an LHRH agonist also caused a decrease in pituitary weight [13].

Table 1. Differences between effects of treatment (*in vitro* and *in vivo*) with the antiprogestin mifepristone (RU486) and with progestins (R5020, megestrol acetate) according to early publications [6,10,11]

		Antiprogestin	Progestin
1.	Inhibition of cellular protein secretion	+	+
	Inhibition of intracellular protein synthesis	+	-
2.	Effect of production on 48 k protein	=	↑
	Effect on production on 52 k protein	=	↓
3.	Effect on ER *in vitro*	↓	↓↓
	Effect on ER *in vivo* (in rat tumours)	↓	↑
	Effect on PR *in vivo* (in rat tumours)	↓↓	↓
4.	Effect on rat organ weights (pituitary, adrenals, ovaries)	↑=	↓
5.	Effect on plasma hormone levels (LH, E2, Prog., ACTH, Cortic., PRL)	↑	↓
6.	Inhibition of E2-stimulated cell growth	+	+
	Inhibition in the absence of E2	+ -	-
7.	Cytostatic effects	+	+
	Cytotoxic effects	+	-
8.	Tumour growth inhibitory effect	+++	++

Effect on Plasma Hormone Levels

In the initial experiments with subcutaneous administration, mifepristone treatment caused increased plasma LH, oestradiol, progesterone and prolactin levels, whereas plasma FSH levels were not significantly affected [9,10]. In subsequent experiments with the three antiprogestins, plasma FSH levels were even slightly suppressed [13,14]. Strikingly, subcutaneous administration of mifepristone (10 mg/kg/day) induced no change in plasma ACTH and corticosterone levels [9, 10], but oral administration of the same dose of the three antiprogestins caused an increase in plasma ACTH and corticosterone levels which was most pronounced for mifepristone. Lower dosages had no clear effect on the pituitary-adrenal function. The addition of tamoxifen and especially an LHRH agonist to treatment with an antiprogestin caused lower plasma oestradiol and progesterone levels than those observed during single treatment with an antiprogestin [13].

Effect on Oestradiol (ER) and Progesterone Receptor (PgR) Levels

The effects of various treatment modalities on cytosolic tumour steroid receptor levels are summarised in Table 2 [13]. Due to its oestrogenic activity tamoxifen caused an increase in PgR synthesis, while megestrol acetate raised ER concentrations. Combination treatment with an antiprogestin (mifepristone) caused nearly complete suppression of PgR levels as measured by ligand binding assay (Scatchard plots). ER levels decreased with all treatments except for high-dose progestin. Interestingly, the combination of an antiprogestin and an antioestrogen suppressed ER levels completely. It should be noted that the treatment modalities that caused the most powerful suppression of both steroid receptors seemed also to induce the best antitumour effects.

Clinical Studies in Postmenopausal Patients with Metastatic Breast Cancer

Antitumour Effects

One of 11 patients showed a partial remission of her lymph-node metastases (58% decrease in tumour size) lasting 5 months; 6 patients showed stable disease of 3-8 months' duration, and 4 showed progressive disease from the start of treatment [12].

Table 2. Effects of different 3-week treatments on cytosolic ER and PgR (fentomoles per mg protein) of rat mammary tumour tissue [13]

Treatment	ER	%	PgR	%
Control	143 ± 75 (23)	100	280 ± 209 (26)	100
TAM (400 μg/kg)	31 ± 26 (19)[a]	22	342 ± 207 (18)	122
RU (10 mg/kg)	47 ± 33 (10)[a]	33	4 ± 13 (14)[a]	1
RU + TAM	2 ± 6 (16)[a]	1	0 (15)[a]	0
LHRH agonist injections (40 μg/kg)	83 ± 53 (18)[a]	58	92 ± 107 (17)[a]	33
LHRH agonist implant	59 ± 32 (4)[b]	41	16 ± 12 (12)[a]	6
RU + LHRH agonist injections	63 ± 33 (17)[a]	44	0 (15)[a]	0
RU + LHRH agonist implant	42 ± 19 (8)[a]	29	4 ± 9 (8)[a]	1

Results are the mean ± SD; the number of determinations is given in parentheses. TAM: Tamoxifen; RU: mifepristone
[a] $P < 0.005$ vs controls
[b] $P < 0.01$ vs controls

In the two clinical studies [12,26] reported so far regarding second or third-line antiprogestin (mifepristone) treatment of a total of 33 patients, 4 patients (12%) showed a partial response, 15 (46%) short-term stable disease and 14 (42%) progressive disease from the start of treatment (Table 3). The beneficial effects were mainly observed in patients with PgR-positive tumours. Strikingly, also some tumours which were or became resistant to treatment with tamoxifen or high-dose progestins showed a response, which makes this new category of drugs of particular interest.

Side Effects

Anorexia and a slight degree of nausea (8 times), tiredness (6 times), malaise and dizziness (4 times) and somnolence (4 times) were relatively frequent complaints. Side effects generally did not occur in the first week of treatment but sometimes after weeks or months of treatment, suggesting that certain plasma levels of mifepristone have to be reached before side effects occur. Ten patients showed a decrease in body weight (mean, 3 kg; range, 0.9-7.5 kg), while one patient had an initial gain in body weight of 5 kg which was followed by a loss of 2 kg without other side effects. We did not observe significant effects on blood pressure. However, one patient using antihypertensive drugs before treatment no longer required antihypertensive treatment after the start of treatment with mifepristone. Two patients had to stop treatment with mifepristone be-

Table 3. Antitumour effects of treatment with the antiprogestin mifepristone (RU 486) in pretreated postmenopausal patients with metastatic breast cancer

	Treatment	No.	PR	MR/NC	PD
1. Romieu et al. (1987)	200 mg/day (third-line)	22	3	9	10
2. Klijn et al. (1989)	200-400 mg/day (second-line)	11	1	6	4
	In total:	33	4 (12%)	15 (46%)	14 (42%)
PgR-positive tumours (all ER+)		7	3	3	1
PgR-negative tumours (5 ER+)		8	0	3	5

Improvement in patients resistant to progestin therapy (1): 3 out of 5
Improvement in patients resistant to tamoxifen therapy (2): 1 out of 11
PR = partial remission; MR = minimal remission; NC = no change; PD = progressive disease

cause of side effects (in the absence of tumour progression). One of these patients was hospitalised because of a grand mal seizure and subcoma under suspicion of cerebral metastases. Treatment with dexamethasone was instituted and mifepristone treatment was stopped. However, no metastases were found on the CT scan of the cerebrum and the patient improved remarkably after 3 days and was dismissed from hospital without any physical complaints. These observations suggest that this complication was induced by mifepristone. In view of the long half-life (approx. 20 h) of mifepristone, the improvement might be related to both excretion of mifepristone and treatment with high-dose dexamethasone, which suppressed the antiglucocorticoid activity of the gradually decreasing plasma levels of mifepristone.

Endocrine Effects

In addition to plasma ACTH, plasma cortisol concentrations showed a highly significant increase during treatment, indicating stimulation of the pituitary-adrenal axis [12]. In contrast to a normal increase in plasma cortisol concentrations by stimulation with synacthen before treatment, there was no significant change in the increased basal cortisol levels by synacthen during mifepristone treatment. Moreover, the increased basal cortisol concentrations could not be suppressed by 1 mg of dexamethasone during mifepristone treatment [12]. Surprisingly, plasma androstenedione and especially plasma oestradiol levels increased significantly during treatment. We found no significant effects on basal and stimulated gonadotropin concentrations, while plasma SHBG concentrations slightly decreased. Plasma oestradiol concentrations were positively correlated with plasma androstenedione ($p<0.05$) and cortisol concentrations ($p<0.01$). Basal prolactin levels did not change during mifepristone treatment, while thyrotropin-releasing hormone-stimulated plasma prolactin concentrations tended to increase, possibly in relation to the increased oestradiol levels [12].
On haematological and biochemical examination a significant increase in the percentage of eosinophilic white blood cells ($p<0.02$) and of plasma creatinine levels ($p<0.05$) was observed, probably as a consequence of the antiglucocorticoid effects of mifepristone [12].

Discussion

In the *in vitro* studies it appeared that the effects of antiprogestin treatment on tumour cell growth are determined by the cell line, culture conditions and dose of the compounds used. With respect to growth inhibition mainly oestrogen-stimulated growth and not basal growth was inhibited. Recently also inhibition of oestrogen-stimulated growth was observed *in vivo* [22]. The best growth inhibitory effect was found in the PgR-rich ER-poor T47D cell line, which was accompanied by a decrease in PgR levels from about 900 to 500 fmol/mg protein (unreported data). Also the oestrogen-stimulated growth of MCF-7 cells was strongly inhibited by antiprogestins, if cultured in human male serum [10]. In serum-free medium high concentrations of mifepristone (10^{-7}-10^{-6}M) caused stimulatory effects on MCF-7 cells as observed with low concentrations of the progestin ORG 2058 [15]. By contrast, high-dose progestin (10^{-6}M) caused the opposite effect, i.e., a slight decrease in cell number, nearly equal to that observed with SFM alone. The stimulatory effect on MCF-7 cells caused by high-dose mifepristone might be explained by a slight intrinsic progestational agonistic activity or by a possible enzymatic conversion of mifepristone to other steroids within the cells. Furthermore, in view of the observation that low concentrations of progestins and in particular very low dosages of oestradiol (10^{-11}-10^{-12} M) can stimulate MCF-cell growth, the possibility of contamination of mifepristone with other steroids has to be considered. When using 1 μM mifepristone, contamination with 0.01-0.0001% of physiological steroids may stimulate cell growth in SFM. On the other hand, we have shown that oestrogen-stimulated growth of breast cancer can be inhibited by antiprogestins. Interestingly, also Jeng and Jordan [27] recently reported the same stimulatory effects of high-dose mifepristone. These stimulatory effects were accompanied by a clear increase in PgR levels, a slight decrease in ER levels, induction of the chloramphenicol acetyltransferase (CAT) reporter gene containing an oestrogen-responsive element (ERE) and a decrease in TGF-B_2 and TGF-B_3. Oestradiol caused similar effects and the growth stimulation of 1 μM mifepristone could be blocked by the antioestrogen ICI 164,384. So, based on their and our experiments, tumour cell growth inhibition was accompanied by a decrease in PgR levels and growth stimulation by an increase. Also *in vivo*, in rats with DMBA-induced mammary tumours, we found a certain relationship between the change in steroid receptor levels and antitumour effects of different treatment modalities [13].

In the rats with DMBA-induced mammary tumours, antiprogestational treatment caused clear tumour growth inhibition and appeared to be more effective than treatment with high-dose progestins or with tamoxifen in spite of high plasma oestradiol and progesterone levels [13,18]. The compound ORG 31710 showed slightly higher antitumour activity than mifepristone and somewhat less antiglucocorticoid effects [14,18]. The mechanism of action of antiprogestational treatment is unclear, but has to be a direct antitumour effect probably via the PgR. Michna, Schneider and coworkers demonstrated that the antiproliferative efficacy of the antiprogestin onapristone is related to its ability to induce terminal differentiation. In contrast to ovariectomy and antioestrogen treatment with tamoxifen, antiprogestin-induced terminal differentiation appeared to be accompanied by down-regulation of tenascin expression (suggested to be a marker of malignant dedifferentiation) in the stromal mesenchyme of DMBA-induced rat mammary tumours [29]. Furthermore, they found that apoptosis of tumour cells during treatment with their antiprogestin was more pronounced than during other endocrine treatment modalities and was accompanied by an accumulation of the tumour cells in the G_0G_1 phase of the cell cycle [22,28].

Most striking was our observation that the addition of tamoxifen to both antiprogestins (mifepristone or ORG 31710) showed additive antitumour effects [12,13,18]. This might be explained by the fact that plasma oestradiol levels were lower during combination therapy or, more probably, by blockade of both ER and PgR (synthesis), resulting in nearly unmeasurable steroid receptor levels. Also *in vitro* additive growth inhibitory effects of mifepristone and tamoxifen have been shown [5]. Recently, Nishino et al. [30] demonstrated additive antitumour effects in several experimental animal models induced by the antiprogestin onapristone in combination with tamoxifen or the pure antioestrogen ICI 164,384.

Also in postmenopausal patients an increase in

MECHANISM OF ACTION OF MIFEPRISTONE (RU486)

DIRECT ANTITUMOUR EFFECTS (via PgR)

INDIRECT ENDOCRINE SIDE EFFECTS

Binding to hypothalamic and pituitary glucocorticoid receptors

↓

Increase CRF and ACTH

↓

Increase cortisol and adrenal androgen secretion

↓

Increase plasma E2 by peripheral conversion of androgens

Fig. 2. Mechanism of action of mifepristone in postmenopausal breast cancer patients

plasma oestradiol levels was observed during mifepristone treatment [12]. However, in contrast to rats where the pituitary-ovarian axis became stimulated, in humans this increase in plasma oestradiol can be explained by stimulation of the pituitary-adrenal axis as based on an increase in plasma ACTH, cortisol and androstenedione levels (Fig. 2). This increase of adrenal androgen secretion, the positive correlation between plasma oestradiol and both cortisol and androstenedione levels, and the observation that the peak value of oestradiol in plasma was reached later than that of cortisol, support the assumption that the rise in plasma oestradiol is mainly derived from peripheral conversion of adrenal androgens by aromatase [12]. The rise in plasma oestradiol levels might explain the relatively short duration of responses observed. Therefore, the combination of an antiprogestin with an antioestrogen or maybe an aromatase inhibitor might be attractive in the treatment of human breast cancer.

In conclusion, antiprogestins form a new category in the endocrine treatment of breast cancer, especially with respect to PgR-positive tumours. Randomised studies comparing the antitumour effects of antiprogestins with those of high-dose progestins or other types of hormonal treatment have to be performed. However, combination treatment with antiprogestins and antioestrogens seems to be of greater interest, aiming at additive growth-inhibitory effects as observed in experimental models. A disadvantage might be the frequent occurrence of side effects caused by the antiglucocorticoid properties of the currently available antiprogestins, but the use of new antiprogestins with less antiglucocorticoid activity which are in an advanced phase of development, should overcome this problem.

Summary

Antiprogestins form a new potential treatment modality for breast cancer. Therefore we performed *in vitro* studies on several breast cancer cell lines and *in vivo* studies in rats with DMBA-induced mammary tumours and in patients with metastatic breast cancer. **In vitro experiments:** antiprogestins can have both growth inhibitory and stimulatory effects *in vitro*, depending on cell lines, culture conditions and dose of the compounds used. Especially the oestrogen-stimulated proliferation of PgR-positive cells is inhibited by antiprogestins in a dose-dependent way. The inhibition caused by ORG 31710 reached a plateau phase at a concentration of 10^{-8}M (74% inhibition), whereas RU 486 did not show a plateau up to 10^{-6}M (53% inhibition). In rats with DMBA-induced mammary tumours, prophylactic treatment with RU 486 resulted in a doubling of the latency period. In rats with existing tumours antiprogestational treatment was slightly more effective than treatment with tamoxifen or progestins. In some experiments the antiprogestin ORG 31710 showed a somewhat more pronounced growth inhibitory effect than the antiprogestins ORG 31806 and RU 486. Most strikingly, combined antiprogestational and antioestrogenic treatment showed additive growth inhibitory effects resulting in clear tumour remissions, in the presence of very strong suppression of ER and PgR levels. Also the growth inhibitory effect of LHRH-agonist treatment was potentiated by antiprogestins. In a preliminary **clinical study** on the efficacy of second-line treatment with RU 486 in 11 postmenopausal patients with breast cancer, we observed one objective response and 6 instances of short-term stable disease. In the two clinical studies reported so far, RU 486 as second or third-line treatment caused a partial response in 12% and stable disease in 46% of 33 patients, particularly in patients with PgR-positive primary tumours. However, clear antiglucocorticoid endocrine and clinical side effects were observed that resulted in very high ACTH, androstenedione and cortisol levels, while consequently plasma oestradiol levels increased due to peripheral aromatisation. In conclusion, treatment with different antiprogestins caused growth inhibitory effects on oestradiol-stimulated PgR-rich tumour cell lines, on rat mammary tumours and in patients with metastatic breast cancer.

Acknowledgements

We thank Roussel-UCLAF (France) and Organon (The Netherlands) for supply of the antiprogestins used in these studies, S.W.J. Lamberts and F.H. de Jong for hormone measurements, Rianne Kalkman for typing the manuscript, and the Dutch Cancer Society for support (grant DDHK 89-6).

REFERENCES

1 Clarke R, Dickson RB and Lippman ME: Hormonal aspects of breast cancer. Growth factors, drugs and stromal interactions. Critical Rev Oncol Hematol 1992 (12):1-23

2 Klijn JGM, Berns PMJJ, Bontenbal M, Alexieva-Figusch J, and Foekens JA: Clinical breast cancer, new developments in selection and endocrine treatment of patients. J Steroid Biochem Molec Biol 1992 (43):211-221

3 Philibert D, Deraedt R, Teutsch G, Tourneminen C and Sakiz E: RU38486 - a new lead for steroidal antihormones. In: Proceedings of the 64th Annual Endocrine Society Meeting, San Francisco, 1982, Abstr 668

4 Bardon S, Vignon F, Chalbos D and Rochefort H: RU486, a progestin and glucococorticoid antagonist, inhibits the growth of breast cancer cells via the progesterone receptor. J Clin Endocrinol Metab 1985 (60):692-697

5 Bardon S, Vignon E, Montcourrier P and Rochefort H: Steroid receptor-mediated cytotoxicity of an antiestrogen and an antiprogestin in breast cancer cells. Cancer Res 1987 (47):1441-1448

6 Gill P, Vignon F, Bardon S, Derocq D and Rochefort H: Difference between R5020 and the antiprogestin RU486 in anti-proliferative effects on human breast cancer cells. Breast Cancer Res Treat 1987 (10):37-45

7 Horwitz KB: The antiprogestin RU38486: receptor-mediated progestin versus antiprogestin actions screened in estrogen-sensitive T47D10 human breast cancer cells. Endocrinology 1985 (116):2236-2245

8 Horwitz KB: The molecular biology of RU486. Is there a role for antiprogestins in the treatment of breast cancer? Endocr Rev 1992 (13):146-163

9 Bakker GH, Setyono-Han B, De Jong FH and Klijn JGM: Mifepristone in treatment of experimental breast cancer in rats. In: Klijn JGM, Paridaens R and Foekes JA (eds) Hormonal Manipulation of Cancer: Peptides, Growth Factors and New (Anti)steroidal Agents. EORTC Monograph Series. Raven Press, New York 1987 Vol 18 pp 39-45

10 Bakker GH, Setyono-Han B, Henkelmann MS, De Jong FH, Lamberts SWJ, Van der Schoot P and Klijn JGM: Comparison of the actions of the antiprogestin mifepristone (RU486), the progestin megestrol acetate, the LHRH-analog buserelin, and ovariectomy in treatment of rat mammary tumors. Cancer Treat Rep 1987 (71):1021-1027

11 Van der Schoot P, Bakker GH and Klijn JGM: Effects of the progesterone antagonist RU486 (mifeprostone) on ovarian activity in the rat. Endocrinology 1987 (121):1375-1382

12 Klijn JGM, De Jong FH, Bakker GH, Lamberts SWJ, Rodenburg CJ and Alexieva-Figusch J: Antiprogestins: a new form of endocrine therapy for breast cancer. Cancer Res 1989 (49):2851-2856

13 Bakker GH, Setyono-Han B, Portengen H, De Jong FH, Foekens JA and Klijn JGM: Endocrine and antitumor effects of combined treatment with an antiprogestin and antiestrogen or luteinizing hormone-releasing hormone agonist in female rats bearing mammary tumors. Endocrinology 1989 (125):1593-1598

14 Bakker GH, Setyono-Han B, Portengen H, de Jong FH, Foekens JA and Klijn JGM: Treatment of breast cancer with different antiprogestins: preclinical and clinical studies. J Steroid Biochem Molec Biol 1990 (37):789-794

15 Bakker GH, Peters HA, Foekens JA and Klijn JGM: Antiprogestin (RU486) and progestin (ORG2058) effects on DNA synthesis in MCF-7 cells. J Cancer Res Clin Oncol 1990 (116: suppl part 1):426 Abstr A.4.116.02

16 Lamberts SWJ, Uitterlinden P, Bons EG and Verleun T: Comparison of the actions of RU38486 and megestrol acetate in the model of a transplantable adrenocorticotropin- and prolactin-secreting rat pituitary tumor. Cancer Res 1985 (45):1015-1019

17 Lamberts SWJ, Koper JW and de Jong FH: The endocrine effects of long-term treatment with mifepristone (RU486). J Clin Endocrinol Metab 1991 (73):187-191

18 Setyono-Han B, Bakker GH, Sander HJ, Foekens JA, Sieuwerts AM, Deckers GH and Klijn JGM: The new antiprogestin ORG31710 significantly inhibits DMBA-induced mammary tumor growth in rats: effects of combination therapy with the aromatase inhibitor ORG 30958 or the antiestrogen tamoxifen. Abstract Book 5th EORTC Breast Cancer Working Conference, Leuven, September 3-6 1991, Abstr A35

19 Schneider MR, Michna H, Nishino Y, and El Etreby MF: Antitumor activity of the progesterone antagonist ZK 98.299 and RU486 in the hormone-dependent MXT mammary tumor model of the mouse and the DMBA- and NMU-induced mammary tumor model of the rat. Eur J Cancer Clin Oncol 1989 (25):691-701

20 Michna H, Schneider MR, Nishino Y, and El Etreby MF: Antitumor activity of the antiprogestins ZK98.299 and RU38486 in hormone dependent rat and mouse mammary tumors: mechanistic studies. Breast Cancer Res Treat 1989 (14):275-288

21 Michna H, Schneider MR, Yishino Y, and El Etreby: The antitumor mechanism of progesterone antagonists is a receptor mediated antiproliferative effect by induction of terminal cell death. J Steroid Biochem 1989 (34):447-453

22 Schneider MR, Michna H, Nishino Y, and El Etreby MF: Antitumor activity and mechanism of action of different antiprogestins in experimental breast cancer models. J Steroid Biochem Molec Biol 1990 (37):783-787

23 Schneider MR, Michna H, Habenicht U-F, Nishino Y, Grill HJ, and Pollow K: The tumour-inhibiting potential of the progesterone antagonist Onapristone in the human mammary carcinoma T61 in nude mice. J Cancer Res Clin Oncol 1992 (118):187-189

24 Foekens JA, Sieuwerts AM, Stuurman-Smeets EMJ, Dorssers LCJ, Berns EMJJ, and Klijn JGM: Pleiotropic actions of suramin on the proliferation of human breast cancer cells in vitro. Int J Cancer 1992 (51): 439-444

25 Bontenbal M, Sieuwerts AM, Klijn JGM, Peters HA, Krijnen HLJM, Sonneveld P, and Foekens JA: Effect of hormonal manipulation and doxorubicin administration on cell cycle kinetics of human breast cancer cells. Br J Cancer 1989 (60): 688-692

26 Romieu G, Maudelonde T, Ulmann A, Pujol H, Grenier J, Cavalie G, Khalaf S and Rochefort H: The antiprogestin RU486 in advanced breast cancer: preliminary clinical trial. Bull Cancer 1987 (74):455-459

27 Jeng MH and Jordan VC: Estrogenic actions of RU486 in estrogen responsive human breast cancer MCF-7 cells. Proceedings of 83rd Annual Meeting of the American Association for Cancer Research, San Diego, May 20-23 1992:282 Abstr 1684

28 Vollmer G, Michna H, Ebert K and Knuppen R: Down-regulation of tenascin expression by antiprogestins during terminal differentiation of rat mammary tumors. Cancer Res 1992 (52):4642-4648

29 Michna H, Nishino Y, Neef G, McGuire WL and Schneider MR: Progesterone antagonists: tumor-inhibiting potential and mechanism of action. J Steroid Biochem Molec Biol 1992 (41):339-348

30 Nishino Y, Schneider MR and Michna H: Enhancement of the antitumor efficacy of an antiprogestin, Onapristone, by combination with antiestrogens. Abstracts Fourth International Congress on Hormones and Cancer, Amsterdam, September 15-19 1991: 227

Immunotherapy of Breast Cancer: Problems and Potential

Joyce Taylor-Papadimitriou

Imperial Cancer Research Fund, 44 Lincoln's Inn Fields, London WC2A 3PX, United Kingdom

Although considerable progress has been made in the clinical management of breast cancer, the impact of present day treatment schedules on survival is less impressive. Furthermore, although pilot studies with novel therapies have been carried out, surgery, radiation therapy, hormonal and chemotherapy in various combinations remain the standard treatment. It seems likely that surgery will continue to be essential for the first-line primary treatment of primary breast cancer, at least in the foreseeable future. However, there is an urgent need to improve the effectiveness of the treatment of metastatic or potentially metastatic disease, since the lack of specificity in cell killing induced by chemotherapy or radiation therapy produces undesirable side effects (with marginal benefits), while induced resistance to the more specific hormone treatment is a common phenomenon. In looking for novel therapies, particularly as an adjuvant to surgery, immunotherapy is an option which is now beginning to be explored. Two reasons why this option may now be a realistic one are that 1) potential target antigens are being identified, and 2) considerable advances have been made in understanding the underlying mechanism involved in antigen presentation and effective recognition of antigen by the various components of the immune system. The possibility of extending immunotherapy to prevention (at least for prevention of recurrence of the disease) is also a real one since ASI (active specific immunotherapy) appears to be unaccompanied by obvious serious side effects.

When a breast cancer, or any other malignant tumour, is detected clinically, the cells making up the tumour have clearly not been rejected by the host's immune system. The implications of this are that even if the tumour does express antigens which can potentially be recognised by some or all of the compartments of the immune system, they are either not being presented effectively or are not being recognised by effector cells. The challenge is therefore two-fold, i.e., to identify relevant antigens and to find a way to present these so that an immune response is generated which is effective in rejecting the tumour cells. In this chapter, we will consider a specific antigen, the polymorphic epithelial mucin (PEM, the product of the MUC1 gene), describe its structure, explain why it may be a candidate target antigen for immunotherapy or preventative vaccination of breast cancer, and discuss the model systems which are available to explore its efficacy as an immunogen. We will also briefly review some of the general problems associated with effective antigen presentation and with tumour cell recognition and what strategies can be adopted to achieve successful tumour rejection.

The Polymorphic Epithelial Mucin (PEM)

Attention was focussed on PEM initially because many antibodies selected for specificity of reaction with epithelial cells or carcinomas were found to react with this molecule [1]. The molecule is therefore extremely immunogenic in the mouse. The gene (MUC1) coding for the core protein of this molecule has been cloned [2-6] and the molecule has been shown to be a transmembrane protein with a cytoplasmic tail of 69 amino acids and a large extracellular domain made up largely of tandem repeats (TR) of 20 amino acids. The TR domain is rich in

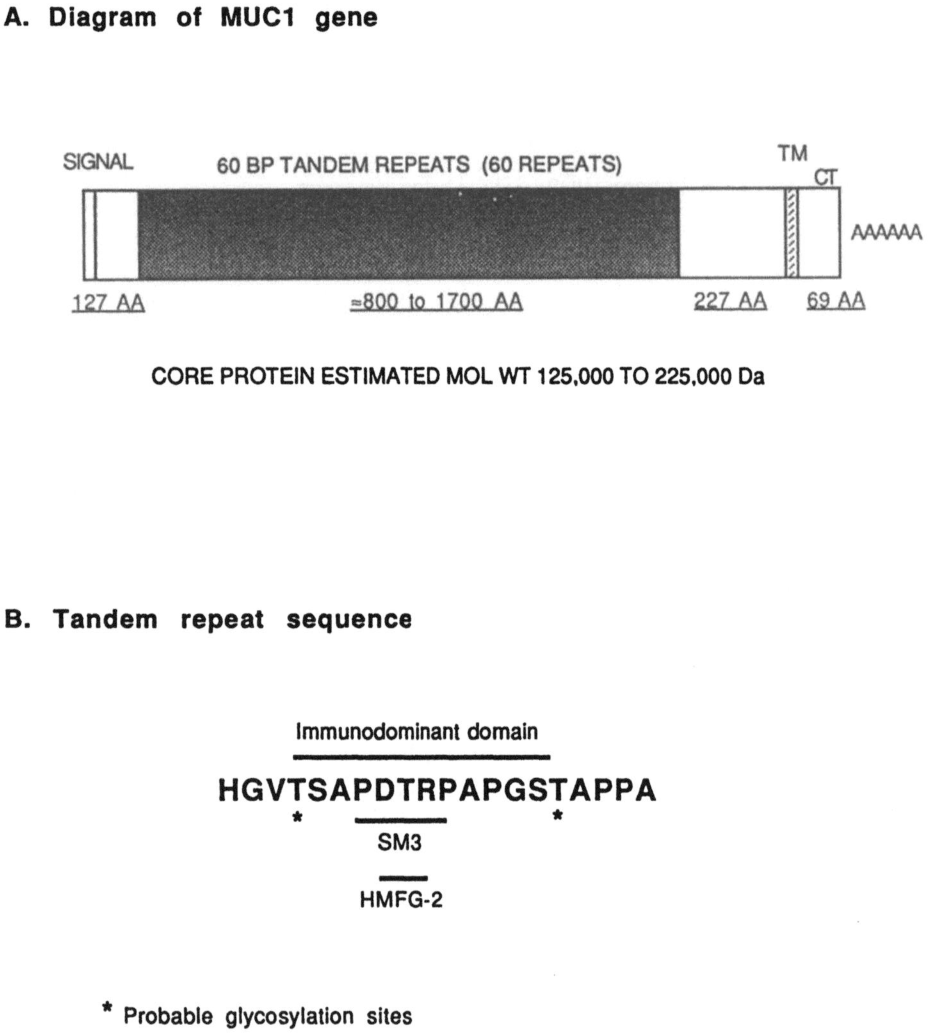

Fig. 1. Diagram of structure of the core protein of PEM

serine, threonine and prolines and serves as a scaffold for the addition of sugars resulting in a very extended rod-like structure (for diagram see Figure 1A). Since the number of tandem repeats can vary with the individual allele, the gene is highly polymorphic. Although PEM, the MUC1 gene product, is expressed on most simple epithelial cells lining glands or ducts, it is dramatically upregulated in the mammary gland at lactation, and in malignancy. The molecule is also aberrantly glycosylated in breast and other carcinomas [7,8], making it antigenically distinct from the normally processed mucin.

Several other human mucin genes (MUC2-4), coding for human mucins found in the lung and gastrointestinal (GI) tract, have subsequently been isolated [9-11] as well as a porcine submaxillary mucin gene [12], genes coding for similar molecules in lower organisms [13,14] and the mouse homologue of the human MUC1 gene [15]. In each case, a large part of the mucin core protein has been found to be made up of tandem repeats, which, though differing in length and sequence, in each case contain high levels of threonine, serine and proline (see Table 1). Although the complete structure of the core proteins of the complex GI and lung mucins has not been elucidated, the data that are available suggest that they are probably not transmembrane molecules. Moreover, they contain cysteine-rich domains [16,17] which probably function to form covalently bonded aggregates. Indeed, PEM may be unique among the mucins in lacking cysteine-rich domains, and in being an intrinsic membrane glycoprotein. It is also the only mucin which has

Table 1. Sequences comprising the tandem repeat units of mucin genes

Name	Source	Sequence
MUC1	Human mammary gland and pancreas	PPAHGVTSAPDTRPAPGSTA
mMUC1	Mouse mammary gland	SPVHSGTSSPATSAPEDSTS
MUC2	Human intestine	PTTTPITTTTTVTPTPTPTGTQT
MUC3	Human intestine	HSTPSFTSSOTTTETTS
MUC4	Human lung	TSSASTGHATPLAPVTA
pMUC?	Porcine salivary gland	GAGPGTTASSVGTETARPSVAGSGTTGTVSGAS GSTGSSSGSPGATGASIGQPETSRISVAGSSGA PAVSSGASQAAGTS
xMUC5	Xenopus	GESTPAPSETT
xMUC6	Xenopus	VPTTPETTT

Sequences contain a high proportion of serines and/or threonines (to which the linkage sugar N-acetylgalactosamine may be attached) and prolines, which provide an extended core protein to allow for up to 90% of the molecule to consist of carbohydrate. The designation of MUC1-4 has been proposed by Gum [5], with the numbers reflecting the order in which the human genes were cloned. The mouse homologue of MUC1 is designated mMUC1 and porcine submaxillary and Xenopus integumentary mucins are designated pMUC and xMUC5 and 6, respectively.

been shown to be overexpressed in carcinomas, the GI mucins being down-regulated in colon carcinomas (2nd International Workshop on Carcinoma-Associated Mucins).

The fact that the MUC1 gene product is a transmembrane molecule which shows increased expression and aberrant glycosylation in cancer makes it an important potential target antigen for antibodies and other components of the immune system.

Aberrant Glycosylation of PEM in Breast Cancer

In studying the profile of reaction of a range of antibodies, some of which are directed to epitopes in the tandem repeat domain, it became clear that the antigenic profile of the cancer-associated mucin was different from the antigenic profile of the mucin produced by the resting or lactating mammary gland [7]. Many of the core protein epitopes detected by mouse monoclonal antibodies are found within an immunodominant domain lying between doublets of serine and threonine which are potential glycosylation sites (Fig. 1) [18,19]. Statistically it is found that only two oligosaccharide side chains are added for each tandem repeat (F.G. Hanisch, personal communication). Recent data following *in vitro* glycosylation with cell extracts suggest that the sites of attachment for these side chains are the threonines flanking the SAPDTRPAPGS sequence (M.A. Hollingsworth, personal communication, see Fig. 1B).

Although the sequence of the MUC1 gene coding for the core protein of PEM is the same in normal and malignant cells [2,20], the length and composition of the carbohydrate side chains vary. A direct analysis of the side chains in milk mucin [21] and in the mucin derived from a breast cancer cell line [22] show that the chains are larger and more complex in the normal mucin than in the breast cancer mucin (see Table 2). The result of the different glycosylation means that novel epitopes appear in the carbohydrate side chains and are unmasked in the core protein of the tumour mucin. The SM3 antibody [7] reacts with such a core protein epitope (see Fig. 1), which is cryptic in the mucin expressed by the normal mammary gland and is selectively exposed in breast cancer [8].

Table 2. Major carbohydrate side chains on PEM

Normal	**Tumour**
(NeuAc2-3)Galβ1-4-GlcNAcb1-6 ↘ GalNAc - ↙ (NeuAc2-3)Galβ1-3	(NeuAc2-6) ↘ GalNAc - ↙ (NeuAc2-3)Galβ1-3
Basic tetrasaccharide and monosialyated products. Also more extended and branched polylactosamine side chains are found and disialylated and fucosylated derivatives.	Basic disaccharide (T) and mono and di-sialylated products, also GalNAc(Tn) and Sialylated Tn.

Antibodies in Imaging and Therapy

A necessary preliminary to attempting to use an antibody for cancer therapy is to demonstrate that the antibody can reach and bind to the tumour cells using radiolabelled antibody. Most of these imaging studies have been done with ovarian cancer patients, since ovarian cancers also overexpress aberrantly glycosylated PEM and the tumours are relatively easy to image, being generally limited to the peritoneal cavity. Thus SM3 antibody has been effectively used to image ovarian cancers [23] and imaging of breast cancers, particularly lymph-node metastases, is now being investigated. Effective imaging of ovarian cancers can also be achieved with antibodies (such as HMFG-2, Fig. 1) which react with epitopes which are also exposed (perhaps at low levels) on the normal mucin, suggesting that *levels* of antigen and tissue topography are an important consideration, since normal PEM-expressing tissues are not imaged.

In attempting to reject tumours using antibody-conjugates to target drugs, toxins or radioactivity, only one element of one compartment of the potential immune response is being manipulated. In spite of this, a pilot study using an Ytrium-labelled antibody to PEM (HMFG-1) [24] as adjuvant therapy in ovarian cancer patients is giving promising results [25]. The important message from these results is that the patients who show increased survival compared to historical controls are those who had minimal residual or undetectable disease following surgery and chemotherapy. Almost certainly any form of immunotherapy is likely to be more effective when the number of malignant cells is small and the cells do not form a solid and possibly impenetrable mass.

Evidence for Immune Recognition of PEM in Cancer Patients

Evidence for immune recognition of the breast cancer mucin was first noted by Finn and colleagues who isolated cytotoxic T cells which killed PEM-expressing cancer cell lines [26,27]. The mechanism involved is unclear, however, since killing is not HLA restricted. This non-HLA restricted killing may arise from the interaction of multiple PEM epitopes with the T cell (not involving the peptide binding groove of the HLA molecule). The core protein epitope (PDTRP, see Fig. 1B) recognised by the antibody SM3 [7,8] is selectively exposed in breast, ovarian and other carcinomas. Moreover, the SM3 antibody has been found to block the killing of PEM-expressing breast cancer cells, suggesting that the core protein epitopes in the vicinity of the PDTRP sequence may be involved in T cell recognition. Recently it has been possible to demonstrate that patients can produce antibodies to PEM, both by detecting their presence in serum (J. Hilgers, personal communication; O. Finn, personal communication) and by isolating and immortalizing B cells producing such antibodies from ovarian cancer patients (A. Rughetti and M. Nuti, personal communication).

Table 3. Possible types of immunogen based on the structure of the cancer-associated polymorphic epithelial mucin

1. Cells expressing the mucin
2. Purified mucin (produced by cancer cells)
3. Recombinant core protein, or different glycoforms produced by transfected cells
4. Peptides, or glycopeptides based on the tandem repeat
5. Recombinant viruses (vaccines, retroviruses)
6. Recombinant BCG
7. Synthetic carbohydrates based on the short carbohydrate side chains found in the cancer-associated mucin (see Table 2)

The range of immunogens based on PEM which could be used to attempt to induce an immune response leading to tumour rejection is wide (Table 3). Trials have begun in breast cancer patients using a synthetic carbohydrate. However, to evaluate the efficacy of the various immunogens, to optimise antigen presentation and to analyse mechanisms involved in tumour rejection, model systems are required.

Rodent Models for Studying Tumour Rejection and Immune Responses to PEM

The TA3-Ha Tumour for Analysis of Carbohydrate Antigens

The shorter carbohydrate side chains which are carried on the core protein of the polymorphic epithelial mucin in many carcinomas are also found on other mucin core proteins in mouse as well as in humans. The mucin expressed by an extremely aggressive mouse mammary adenocarcinoma TA3-Ha also carries these side chains, and this mouse model has been used effectively to analyse the efficacy of synthetic carbohydrates as immunogens [28,29]. Antibody responses to T (Gal1-3GalNAc) coupled to KLH have been seen in immunised mice and inhibition of tumour growth was seen even when the immunogen was administered after the tumour cells were injected [28]. Ovine submaxillary mucin (carrying multiple sialylated Tn epitopes, i.e., NeuAc 2-6GalNAc) and its desialylated product, have also been found to be effective in both stimulating an immune response and in inhibiting tumour growth in this system [29]. Although cellular responses to carbohydrates are not well studied, they have been shown to induce delayed type hypersensitivity (DTH) responses and T cell proliferation in immunised mice [28,29]. The phase 1 trial in breast cancer patients which has begun in Canada [30] uses synthetic Sialyl Tn coupled to KLH (Keyhole Limpet Hemocyanin) as immunogen since there is some indication that the expression of this particular epitope may be more specifically associated with metastatic cells.

Syngeneic Model System Using a Mouse Mammary Tumour Cell Line Transfected with the Human MUC1 Gene

A syngeneic model for comparing the efficacy of immunogens based on PEM was developed by introducing the MUC1 gene into the mouse mammary epithelial tumour cell line 410.4 [30]. Expression of the human PEM resulted in a reduced growth of tumours in Balb/c/c mice at low inoculum, but tumours did develop provided sufficient cells (10^5) were injected. A variety of immunogens can be used (see Table 3) and to date we have been able to show that inhibition of tumour growth can be achieved by pre-immunisation with transfected cells [30]; peptides based on the tandem repeat sequence of PEM [31]; and a recombinant vaccinia virus carrying the MUC1 gene (J. Lewis, H. Stauss, E.N. Lalani, T. Taylor-Papadimitriou, unpublished observations).

Transgenic Mice Expressing the Human MUC1 Gene

To look at immune responses in a host where the human PEM is expressed as a self antigen, a transgenic mouse has been developed. The MUC1 gene is compact (Fig. 2), being closely flanked 3' by the thrombospondin 3 gene [32] and 5' by a gene giving a large transcript (13 kb) in most tissues (S.J. Gendler and T. Duhig, personal communication). Perhaps not surpris-

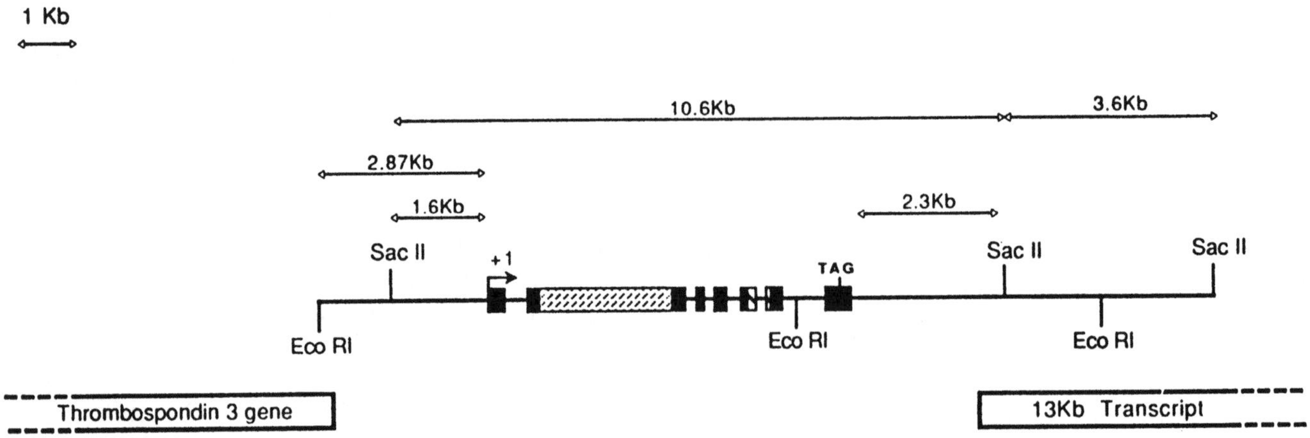

Fig. 2. Diagram of MUC1 gene and flanking sequences

ingly, therefore, we have been able to obtain accurate tissue-specific expression in a transgenic mouse using a 10.6 kb fragment of genomic DNA containing only 1.5 kb of 5' sequence and 2.3 kb of 3' sequence [34]. In humans, the MUC1 gene is expressed largely by simple epithelial cells, and the same distribution (as determined by staining with antibodies specific for the human PEM) is seen in the transgenic mouse. These mice therefore provide an appropriate model for toxicity testing of antibodies or antigens related to the human PEM. It is also possible to look at humoral responses to PEM-based immunogens and to examine T cell proliferative responses *in vitro*. Since the mice are hybrid, it will be necessary to backcross on to a single strain in order to be able to analyse H_2 restricted cytotoxic T cell responses. Cytotoxic T cell responses which are not H_2 restricted can, however, be analysed. We are also presently attempting to obtain a transgenic strain which spontaneously develops mammary or other epithelial tumours.

Antigen Presentation

Classically, antigens are administered with adjuvant, which in a general way acts to induce a more effective immune response. In this context the idea of using a recombinant BCG vaccine [35] expressing PEM is particularly attractive, since BCG has been widely administered to humans as an anti-TB vaccine and attempts to make such a construct are beginning. In addition to using a non-specific adjuvant, there are at least two other approaches which can be used to improve antigen presentation which are important and should be tried. The first relates to the requirement for co-stimulation of T lymphocytes. The second to supplying a specific lymphokine along with the antigen to enhance T cell proliferation.

The B7/BB1 Molecule in Co-Stimulation of T Lymphocytes

It is known that molecules which interact with the antigen-specific T cell receptor (peptides bound to MHC, antibodies to the receptor, lectins) cannot alone stimulate IL-2 production and T cell proliferation which requires additional signals. The additional signals appear to be generated by the interaction of molecules expressed on the lymphocyte (CD28 or CTLA-4) with the B7/BB1 (hereafter referred to as B7) molecule expressed on antigen presenting cells [36-38]. CD28 and CTLA-4 may interact cooperatively to give maximum B7 binding, and are probably derived from the same ancestral gene [39]. Carcinoma cells, which would be expected to be the antigen presenting cells in the cancer patient, do not express B7, and would not therefore be co-stimulating the T cell, even if the cell receptor is engaged. Moreover, engagement of the receptor in the absence of co-stimulation (and the concomitant inadequacy of IL-2 production) results in the production of inhibitors which block further proliferation of the T cell [40]. The T cell is then said to be in a state of anergy, which involves a block in IL-2 production and in responsiveness to IL-4. An exciting development recently reported by Peter Linsley and colleagues is that if the B7 gene is transfected into and expressed in tumour cells, the transfectants are rejected whereas the original tumour was not [41]. The mechanism of rejection appears to depend on direct activation of CD8+ cytotoxic T cells which can, with co-stimulation, make their own IL-2, and do not depend on effective stimulation of CD4+ helper T cells. Of great importance is the observation that the B7+ cells could cause regression of B7- tumour cells at distant sites, showing that B7 is not required for cell killing. These observations introduce the possibility of a new treatment modality in immunotherapy which involves transfecting B7 into the cell used for immune stimulation.

Using autologous tumour cells transfected with B7 is an expensive and labour-intensive form of individual therapy. However, if, as is suggested from the results of Finn and colleagues, the response to PEM is not HLA restricted, it may be possible to use one allogeneic cell line expressing PEM and B7. Using transfected cells as immunogens would also allow the introduction of yet another aid to antigen presentation, i.e., the co-expression of a lymphokine.

Expression of Lymphokines in Cells Used as Immunogen

Mouse models have been used to examine the effect of injecting irradiated tumour cells expressing various lymphokines (e.g., interferons, interleukins, GM-CSF) on subsequent tumour development in mice challenged, not only with the transfected cells, but with the tumour cells not expressing the lymphokine [42,43]. These studies have renewed enthusiasm for the concept of cancer vaccines. In the study reported by Dranoff et al., a variety of cytokine genes were introduced using retroviruses into B16 melanoma cells. These investigators found that irradiated cells expressing GM-CSF stimulated potent, long lasting and specific anti-tumour immunity which depended on CD4+ and CD8+ T cells. The results could have important implications for the clinical use of genetically engineered tumour cells as vaccines. Retroviruses ensure that the gene may be introduced into a large number of the cells, and the possibility of using irradiated cells avoids the obvious problems which may arise with the use of live tumour cells. Another possibility is to use a fusion protein which carries the antigenic determinant and the functional lymphokine. Where a specific peptide has been identified as being recognised by cytotoxic T cells, this can also be coupled to a T helper epitope. The bifunctional peptide could then be presented by antigen presenting cells (which do express B7) to both helper and cytotoxic T cells and the expression of lymphokines necessary for T cell proliferation would be induced.

Tumour Cells as Targets

Relevance of HLA class 1 expression

Although it is not clear which of the immune responses play an important role in killing human breast cancer cells, the data from animal models suggest that CD8+ cytotoxic T cells are likely to be involved. In this case, the antigen is generally presented as a peptide (produced inside the antigen presenting cell) in the groove of the HLA class I molecule expressed on most cells of the body (for review see ref. 44). Where tumour cells are presenting the antigen to the T cell receptor, problems related to HLA expression may be encountered. Firstly, antigen presentation is likely to be HLA- restricted since the HLA-peptide interaction is specific for a particular allele and the antigen may be presented by only some HLA alleles. Secondly, many cancers lose expression of the HLA-class 1 molecules and therefore cannot present antigens at all to the T cells [45]. In this case, even if a strong immune response is generated, killing will not occur - at least not through an HLA-dependent mechanism. Selection for HLA-class I negative tumour cells may be used as an argument to support the idea of immune surveillance, which the tumour in this way has eluded.

In the case of the PEM antigen, the cytotoxic T cells which have been isolated from breast cancer patients, do not appear to be HLA restricted in their killing of targets, and indeed can kill PEM-expressing HLA-class I negative cells [26,27]. They do, however, only kill targets expressing the aberrantly glycosylated mucin. The lack of requirement for HLA could be an enormous advantage and argues for using immunogens based on PEM in immunotherapy of breast cancers.

Another way to avoid the requirement for HLA class I expression by tumours is to construct bispecific antibodies which show a specific reaction with both a target antigen and the CD3 T cell receptor. The antibody then brings the tumour cell close to the T cell without requiring the HLA class I molecule. Clinical studies are in progress using a bispecific antibody reactive with an ovarian cancer antigen, and preliminary results indicate that responses can be obtained even with late-stage patients (M. Colnaghi, personal communication).

Conclusions

Until now, attempts to mobilise the immune system for rejection of breast cancers have used non-specific stimuli such as BCG or IL-2, and these trials have met with little success. Identification of specific target antigens, together with the developing understanding of the mechanisms involved in antigen presentation and in tumour cell killing, now allows the possibility of manipulating the immune system in a more specific and directed manner. The next few years should see trials based on this approach being launched and in this writer's opinion, we can expect some exciting results.

REFERENCES

1 Burchell J and Taylor-Papadimitriou J: Antibodies to human milk fat globule molecules. Cancer Invest 1989 (17):53-61
2 Gendler SJ, Lancaster CA, Taylor-Papadimitriou J, Duhig T, Peat, N, Burchell J, Pemberton L, Lalani E-N and Wilson D: Molecular cloning and expression of the human tumour-associated polymorphic epithelial mucin. J Biol Chem 1990 (265):15286-15293
3 Ligtenberg M, Vos H, Gennissen A and Hilkens J: Episialin, a carcinoma-associated mucin, is generated by a plymorphic gene encoding splice variants with alternative amino termini. J Biol Chem 1990 (265):5573-5578
4 Wreschner DH, Hareuveni M, Tsarfaty I et al: Human epithelial tumor antigen cDNA sequences. Eur J Biochem 1990 (189):463-473
5 Siddiqui J, Abe M, Hayes D, Shani E, Yunis E and Kufe D: Isolation and sequencing of a cDNA coding for the human DF3 breast carcinoma-associated antigen. Proc Natl Acad USA 1988 (85):2320-2323
6 Lan M, Batra S, Qi W-N, Metzgar R and Holingsworth M: Cloning and sequencing of a human pancreatic tumour mucin cDNA. J Biol Chem 1990 (265):15294-15299
7 Burchell J, Gendler SJ, Taylor-Papadimitriou J, Girling A, Lewis A, Millis R and Lamport D: Development and characterisation of breast cancer reactive monoclonal antibodies directed to the core protein of the human milk mucin. Cancer Res 1987 (47):5476-5482
8 Girling JR, Bartkova J, Burchell J, Gendler S, Gillett C and Taylor-Papadimitriou J: A core protein epitope of the polymorphic epithelial mucin detected by the monoclonal antibody SM-3 is selectively exposed in a range of primary carcinomas. Int J Cancer 1989 (43): 1072-1076
9 Gum JR, Byrd J, Hicks J, Toribara N, Lamport D and Kim Y: Molecular cloning of human intestinal mucin cDNAs. J Biol Chem 1989 (264):6480-6487
10 Gum JR, Hicks J, Swallow D et al: Molecular cloning of cDNAs derived from a novel human intestinal mucin gene. Biochem Biophys Res Commun 1990 (171):407-415
11 Porchet N, Van Cong N, Dufosse J, Audie JP, Guyonnet-Duperat V, Gross MS, Denis C, Degand P, Bernheim A and Aubert JP: Molecular cloning and chromosomal localization of a novel human tracheo-bronchial mucin cDNA containing tandemly repeated sequences of 48 base pairs. Biochem Biophys Res Commun 1991 (175):414-422
12 Timpte C, Eckhardt A, Abernethy J and Hill R: Porcine submaxillary gland apomucin contains tandemly repeated, identical sequences of 81 residues. J Biol Chem 1988 (263):1081-108
13 Hoffman W: A new repetitive protein from *Xenopus laevis* skin highly homologous to pancreatic spasmolytic polypeptide. J Biol Chem 1988 (263):7686-7690
14 Probst JC, Gertzen E-M and Hoffman W: An integumentary mucin (FIM-B.I) from *Xenopus laevis* homologous with von Willebrand factor. Biochem 1990 (29):6240-6244
15 Spicer AP, Parry G, Patton S and Gendler SJ: Molecular cloning and analysis of the mouse homologue of the tumor-associated mucin, MUC1, reveals conservation of potential O-glycosylation sites, transmembrane and cytoplasmic domains and a loss of minisatellite-like polymorphism. J Biol Chem 1991 (266):15099-15109
16 Eckhardt AE, Timpte CS, Abernethy JL, Zhao Y and Hill RL: Porcine submaxillary mucin contains a cysteine-rich, carboxyl-terminal domain in addition to a highly repetitive, glycosylated domain. J Biol Chem 1991 (266):9678-9686
17 Gum JR, Hicks JW, Toribara NW, Rothe EM, Lagace RE and Kim YS: The human MUC2 intestinal mucin has cysteine-rich subdomains located both upstream and downstream of its central repetitive region. J Biol Chem 1992 (267):21375-21383
18 Burchell J, Taylor-Papadimitriou J, Boshell M, Gender SJ and Duhig T: A short sequence within the amino acid tandem repeat of a cancer associated mucin, contains immunodominant epitopes. Int J Cancer 1989 (44):691-696
19 Taylor-Papadimitriou J: Report on the First International Workshop on Carcinoma-Associated Mucins. Int J Cancer 1991 (49):1-5
20 Lancaster C, Peat N, Duhig T, Wilson D, Taylor-Papadimitriou J and Gendler S: Structure and expression of the human polymorphic epithelial mucin gene: an expressed VNTR unit. Biochem Biophys Res Commun 1990 (173):1019-1029
21 Hanish FG, Uhlenbruck G, Peter-Katalinic J, Egge H, Dabrowski J and Dabrowski U: Structures of neutral O-linked polylactosaminoglycans on human skim milk mucins. A novel type of linearly extended poly-N-acetyl-lactosamine backbones with Galb(1-4) GlcNAcb(1-6) repeating units. J Biol Chem 1989 (265):872-883
22 Hull SR, Bright A, Carraway KL, Abe M, Hayes DF and Kufe DW: Oligosaccharide differences in the DF3 sialomucin antigen from normal human milk and the BT-20 human breast carcinoma cell line. Cancer Commun 1989 (1):261-267
23 Granowska M, Mather SJ, Jobling T, Naeem M, Burchell J, Taylor-Papadimitriou J, Shepherd J and Britton KE: Radiolabelled stripped mucin, SM3, monoclonal antibody for immunoscintigraphy of ovarian tumours. Int J Biol Markers 1990 (5):89-96
24 Burchell J, Durbin H and Taylor-Papadmitriou J: Complexity of expression of antigenic determinants recognised by monoclonal antibodies HMFG-1 and HMFG-2, in normal and malignant human mammary epithelial cells. J Immunol 1983 (131):508-513
25 Hird V, Snook D, Dhokia B, Sutter WP, Mears C, Stewart JSW, Mason P, Lambert H and Epenetos AA: Adjuvant therapy of ovarian cancer with radiolabelled monoclonal antibody. Br J Canc 1993 (in press)
26 Barnd DL, Lan MS, Metzgar RS and Fin OJ: Specific, major histocompatibility complex-unrestricted recognition of tumor-associated mucins by human cytotoxic T cells. Proc Natl Acad Sci USA 1989 (86):7159-7164
27 Jerome KR, Barnd KL, Bendt KM, Boyer CM, Taylor-Papadimitriou J, McKenzie IFC, Bast Jr. RC and Finn OJ: Cytotoxic T-lymphocytes derived from

patients with breastadenocarcinoma recognise an epitope present on the protein core of a mucin molecule preferentially expressed by malignant cells. Cancer Res 1991 (51):2908-2916

28 Fung PYS, Madej M, Koganty R and Longnecker BM: Active specific immunotherapy of a murine mammary adenocarcinoma using a synthetic tumor-associated glycoconjugate. Cancer Res 1990 (50):4308

29 Singhal A, Fohn M and Hakomori S: Induction of a-N-Acetylgalactosamine-O-serine/threonine (Tn) antigen-mediated cellular immune response for active immunotherapy in mice. Cancer Res 1991 (51): 1406-1414

30 Longenecker BM, Reddish M, Koganty R, and MacLean GD: Immune responses of mice and human breast cancer patients following immunization with synthetic sialyl-Tn conjugated to KLH plus DETOX™ adjuvant. Proc NY Acad Sci 1993 (in press).

31 Lalani EN, Berdichevsky F, Boshell M, Shearer M, Wilson D, Stauss H, Gendler SJ and Taylor-Papadimitriou J: Expression of the gene coding for a human mucin in mouse mammary tumour cells can affect their tumorigenicity. J Biol Chem 1991 (266):15420-15426

32 Ding L, Lalani E-N, Reddish M, Koganty R, Wong T, Samuel J, Yacyshyn MB, Meikle A, Fung PYS, Taylor-Papadimitriou J and Longnecker BM: Immunogenicity of synthetic peptides related to the core peptide sequence encoded by the human MUC1 mucin gene: effect of immunization on the growth of murine mammary adenocarcinoma cells transfected with the human MUC1 gene. J Cancer Immunol Immunotherapy 1993 (in press)

33 Vos HL, Devarayalu Y, de Vries and Bornstein P: Thrombospondin 3 (Thbs3), a new member of the thrombospondin gene family. J Biol Chem 1992 (267):12192-12196

34 Peat N, Gendler SJ, Lalani E-N, Duhig T and Taylor-Papadimitriou J: Tissue-specific expression of a human poymorphic epithelial mucin (MUC1) in transgenic mice. Cancer Res 1992 (52):1954-1960

35 Aldovini A and Young RA: Humoral and cell-mediated immune responses to live recombinant BCG-HIV vaccines. Nature 1991 (351):479-482

36 Linsley PS, Clark EA and Ledbetter JA: T-cell antigen CD28 mediates adhesion with B cells by interacting with activation antigen B7/BB-1. Proc Natl Acad Sci USA 1990 (87):5031-5035

37 Linsley PS, Brady W, Grosmaire L, Aruffo A, Damle NK and Ledbetter JA: Binding of the B cell activation antigen B7 to CD28 costimulates T cell proliferation and interleukin 2 mRNA accumulation. J Exp Med 1991 (173):721-730

38 Linsley PS, Brady W, Urnes M, Grosmaire LS, Damle NK and Ledbetter JA: CTLA-4 is a second receptor for the B cell activation antigen B7. J Exp Med 1991 (174):561-569

39 Harper K, Balzano C, Rouvier E, Mattei M-G, Luciani M-F and Golstein P: CTLA-4 and CD28 activated lymphocyte molecules are closely related in both mouse and human as to sequence, message expression, gene structure and chromosomal location. J Immun 1991 (147):1037-1044

40 Schwartz RH: A cell culture model for T lymphocyte clonal anergy. Science 1990 (248):1349-1356

41 Chen L, Ashe S, Brady WA, Hellstrom I, Hellstrom KE, Ledbetter JA, McGowan P and Linsley PS: Costimulation of antitumor immunity by the B7 counter receptor for the T lymphocyte molecules CD28 and CTLA-4. Cell 1992 (71):1093-1102

42 Golumbek PT, Lazenby AJ, Levitsky HI, Jaffee LM, Karasuyama H, Baker M and Pardoll DM: Treatment of established renal cancer by tumor cells engineered to secrete interleukin-4. Science 1991 (254):713-716

43 Dranoff G, Jaffee E, Lazenby A, Golumbek P, Levitsky H, Brose K, Jackson V, Hamada H, Pardoll D and Mulligan RC: Vaccination with irradiated tumor cells engineerd to secrete murine GM-CSF stimulates potent, specific and long lasting anti-tumor immunity. (submitted)

44 McMichael A: Cytotoxic T lymphocytes specificity, surveilance and escape. Adv Canc Res 1992 (59):227-244

45 Smith MEF, Marsh SGE, Bodmer JG, Gelsthorpe K and Bodmer WF: Loss of HLA-A,A,B,C allele products and lymphocute function-associated antigen 3 in colorectal neoplasia. Proc Natl Acad Sci USA 1989 (86):5557-5561

Adjuvant Chemo-Endocrine Therapy

Manfred Kaufmann

Universitäts-Frauenklinik, Voßstraße 9, 69115 Heidelberg, Germany

Both chemotherapy and endocrine therapy are established treatment modalities in advanced [1-3] and primary [4-7] breast cancer. Their mode of action, antitumour efficacy and side effects are different. The rationale for combining the two modalities is, therefore, to achieve higher response rates, longer periods to progression, longer disease-free intervals and longer and better survival. Since breast cancer is a very heterogeneous disease, additive or synergistic effects on tumour cells are to be expected.

The anticancer effects induced by cytotoxic treatment are mainly direct effects on the tumour cells, whereas endocrine therapy primarily changes the endocrine milieu of the tumour patient (host). Endocrine treatment also affects tumour cells in an indirect way which is often receptor dependent. Different spectra of toxicity favour the simultaneous application of the two modalities; however, they may sometimes interact in a negative way [8,9].

Clinical data from studies on advanced breast cancer which compared chemo-endocrine combinations to either endocrine or chemotherapy alone showed an advantage in terms of remission rates from the chemo-endocrine combination. This initial advantage, however, never resulted in a survival benefit [1].

Chemo-endocrine therapy may be more effective as adjuvant treatment due to the reduced tumour mass of the primary tumour, to different chemosensitivity, e.g., different amounts of hormone-receptor positive or negative tumour cells, and possibly to the positive "side effects" of antioestrogens.

Currently used endocrine manoeuvres or drugs for palliative and adjuvant therapy are listed in Table 1. In palliative treatment of advanced breast cancer surgical ovariectomy can be replaced by medical castration using GnRH analogues in premenopausal patients [10] and this can be transferred to the adjuvant setting. Antioestrogens (tamoxifen) are effective in pre- and postmenopausal patients.

Table 1. Endocrine procedures to achieve antitumour effects in metastatic and primary breast cancer according to menopausal status

Menopausal status	**Procedure**	**Effect**
Premenopausal	oophorectomy	direct ablation
Premenopausal	GnRH analogues	indirect suppression, direct tumour effect by binding sites
Premenopausal/ postmenopausal	tamoxifen	as **antagonist** direct antitumour effect as **agonist** stimulating effect (endocrine resistance)

Table 2. Side effects of tamoxifen which may influence survival in primary breast cancer

Reduction of cardiovascular events
Reduction of cholesterol (LDL)
Reduction of bone loss
Reduction of contralateral breast cancer
Induction of endometrial cancer

In contrast to cytotoxic anticancer drugs, antioestrogens may show "positive" side effects [11,12] which may influence survival in patients treated with adjuvant therapy (Table 2). Besides data on direct tumour effects, little knowledge has been yielded by the studies that analysed changes in the endocrine milieu due to adjuvant endocrine or cytotoxic treatment alone or in combination (Table 3). It has clearly been demonstrated that ovarian ablation, tamoxifen or cytotoxic adjuvant treatment modalities have different effects on LH, FSH, oestradiol and progesterone blood levels. Combinations of either endocrine therapies alone or chemo-endocrine treatment can induce quite diverging hormone levels. There is little information available on chemo-endocrine therapy combinations.

Many studies have attempted to improve the results by combining chemotherapy and endocrine therapy based on the theoretically demonstrated advantages. Various clinical trials have addressed diverse questions about the role of combined chemotherapy and endocrine therapy. However, most of these trials suffer from small sample sizes and failure to stratify patients on the basis of menstrual status or established prognostic factors. Therefore reliable data can only be obtained by analysing the world-wide overview of the Early Breast Cancer Trialists' Collaborative Group (EBCTCG) published in detail in 1992 [5].

Table 3. Influence of adjuvant systemic therapies on LH, FSH, E_2, and progesterone blood levels in women with primary breast cancer

	LH	FSH	E2	Progesterone
Premenopause				
Ovarian ablation	↑	↑	↓	↓
GnRH	↓	↓	↓	↓
Tam	↑	↑	↑	↑
Chemotherapy (amenorrhoea induced)	↑	↑	↓	↓
Postmenopause				
Tam	↓	↓	-	-
Chemotherapy	-	-	-	-
Chemoendocrine therapy (CTX + Tam)	?	?	?	?
Premenopause	(↑)	(↑)	(↑)	(-)
Postmenopause	(↓)	(↓)	-	(-)

↑ = increase; ↓ = decrease

Table 4. EBCTCG overview [5]: Typical reduction % in annual odds of recurrence or prior death (R) and death from any cause (D)

	No. pts.		R		D	
	<50	50+	<50	50+	<50	50+ years
CTX vs. nil	2976	3745	37	22	27	14
Tam vs. nil	2216	13,114	27	30	(17)	19
CTX + Tam vs. Tam	386	3932	(32)	26	(-6)	10
Tam + CTX vs. CTX	6362	8148	7	28	3	20
Ov vs. nil	878	-	(30)	-	(28)	-
CTX + Ov vs. CTX	939	-	(21)	-	(19)	-

( ) = SD ≥ 9; CTX = polychemotherapy; Tam = tamoxifen; Ov = ovarian ablation

EBCTCG - Overview of Adjuvant Therapy of Breast Cancer - Chemo-Endocrine Therapies

Recently the EBCTCG has reviewed almost all randomised trials on adjuvant therapy for primary breast cancer conducted world-wide. This overview found that highly significant reductions in the annual rates of recurrence and death were produced by chemotherapy (recurrence 21 ± 2 % SD; mortality 11 ± 2 % SD), castration below age 50 (recurrence 26 ± 6 % SD; mortality 25 ± 7 % SD) and tamoxifen (recurrence 25 ± 2 % SD; mortality 17 ± 2 % SD) [5].

Polychemotherapy appears to be more active in young patients (<50 years of age), whereas endocrine therapy (tamoxifen, given e.g. for 2-5 years) appears to be more active in older patients (50+, postmenopausal). Ovarian ablation was active only in premenopausal women. The overview also addresses questions concerning the role of combined endocrine and chemotherapy. How can treatment results be improved? Is chemo-endocrine therapy more effective in the adjuvant setting compared to either therapy alone? Is chemotherapy plus endocrine treatment (tamoxifen, castration or both) superior to chemotherapy alone in premenopausal patients? Is tamoxifen in combination with chemotherapy of benefit in all postmenopausal patients?

In Table 4 typical reductions (%) in the annual odds of recurrence and death are shown for cytotoxic and endocrine therapy or their combinations in separate patient groups (<50 or 50+ years of age). For women under 50 it has not been established that combined tamoxifen-cytotoxic therapy is any better than either treatment alone. However, this may also be due to the small number of patients studied so far. Chemotherapy plus ablation seems to be superior to chemotherapy alone in premenopausal patients.

The proportional reduction in annual odds of death (%) in stage II breast cancer is given in Table 5 for pre- and postmenopausal patients treated with chemotherapy, ablation, tamoxifen or tamoxifen/chemotherapy.

The combination of tamoxifen plus chemotherapy resulted in some additive benefit in comparison to either modality alone (Table 6). For women aged 50-69 indirect comparison shows that chemotherapy plus tamoxifen is significantly better than chemotherapy alone both for recurrence and mortality and better than tamoxifen alone for recurrence. Indirect estimates of the effects of tamoxifen with or without chemo-

Table 5. EBCTCG overview [5]: Proportional reduction in annual odds of death % (SD) in stage II breast cancer

	<50		50+ years	
CTX	25	(5)	12	(4)
Ov	28	(9)	-	
Tam	-		20	(2)
CTX + Tam	-		30	(5)

Table 6. EBCTCG overview [5]: Indirectly estimated effects of typical reduction % in annual odds of recurrence or prior death (R) and death from any cause (D)

	R		D	
	<50	50+	<50	50+ years
Tam + CTX to Tam	-	48	-	27
CTX + Tam to CTX	-	44	-	31
CTX + Ov to CTX	40-50?	-	30-40?	-

therapy suggest that tamoxifen may be less effective for women under 50 if chemotherapy is given simultaneously. The combination of chemotherapy plus ablation in comparison to chemotherapy alone, however, resulted in an impressive additive benefit both for reduction of recurrence and death.

Table 7 summarises the survival benefit of single therapies and possible treatment combinations in pre and postmenopausal patients. Combined chemo and endocrine therapy is most effective in premenopausal patients if the endocrine treatment is ablation and tamoxifen shows the best results in postmenopausal patients. However, there is a need for more randomised trials focussing on all these direct comparisons including different duration and timing of tamoxifen or GnRH-analogues instead of surgical castration to optimise adjuvant therapy.

Table 7. Summary of survival benefit by different adjuvant systemic treatments in pre- and postmenopausal women

Treatment	Premenopausal	Postmenopausal
CTX	++	+
Tam	+	++
Ov	++	-
CTX + Tam	-	+
Tam + CTX	+	+++
CTX + Ov	+++	-
Ov + Tam ± CTX	?	-
GnRH analogues	?	-

CTX = polychemotherapy; Tam = tamoxifen; Ov = ovarian ablation

For premenopausal women there is some evidence that the duration of tamoxifen treatment was shorter [5] and therefore not comparable to the results obtained in postmenopausal patients. In many instances data are also lacking as to whether tamoxifen was followed by chemotherapy or given simultaneously.

1992 International Consensus Panel Recommendations for Risk-Adapted Adjuvant Therapy

The 10 and 15-year overview analysis influenced the treatment recommendations outside clinical trials that were established at the St. Gallen Conference in February 1992 [13]. Treatment recommendations have been made for node-negative and node-positive patients. Node-negative patients were divided into minimal, low, and high-risk groups. Combined chemo and endocrine therapy was suggested for node-negative high-risk and node-positive patients (Table 8).

Table 8. 1992 International Consensus Panel Recommendations for node-negative (N-) high-risk and node-positive (N+) primary breast cancer

N- high risk; N+	ER-	ER+
Premenopausal	CTX	CTX ± Tam.
Postmenopausal	CTX ± Tam	Tam ± CTX
Elderly (70+ yrs)	CTX (if tolerable) or Tam	Tam

The selection of therapy was made according to oestrogen receptor and menopausal status or age. There is an evident need for further randomised trials to make sure that the combination of chemo-endocrine treatment has greater absolute benefits than either chemotherapy or endocrine therapy alone.

Future Aspects

New treatment modalities in prospective randomised trials should be based on the worldwide EBCTCG overview update. In addition, innovative pilot studies may lead to further progress.

In the next generation of randomised trials ovarian ablation (e.g., medical castration by GnRH analogues) versus cytotoxic treatment versus both therapies have to be tested in premenopausal patients. In postmenopausal women tamoxifen will be the standard treatment in comparison to combined chemo-endocrine therapy. Only few data exist concerning elderly women where tamoxifen and perhaps biological response modifiers may play an important role in the future. It is also unclear today what the optimal combination and sequence of chemo-endocrine therapies is. Further studies will elaborate the optimal endocrine and cytotoxic therapies. The interaction of different treatment modalities will include surgery, radiotherapy and systemic treatments. The mode of timing adjuvant chemo-endocrine therapy and the aims of different timing modalities are shown in Table 9. Combined chemo-endocrine therapy can be simultaneous, sequential, intermittent, and alternating.

Table 9. Mode and aim of timing of adjuvant chemo-endocrine therapies

Mode of timing	Main aim of timing
Simultaneous	additive effect
Sequential	against heterogeneity
Intermittent	withdrawal effect
Alternating	reinduction to overcome drug resistance

We also need further and more precise definitions of the hormonal situation of breast cancer patients which includes circulating oestrogen blood levels, as well as information on the influence of such matters as hormone replacement therapy. With this knowledge and with the help of current and new prognostic factors better selection of patients for adjuvant therapy will be possible. New predictive factors will select patients more appropriately for adjuvant chemo and/or endocrine therapies [14,15]. In addition, new endocrine drugs will have to be considered in adjuvant trial designs.

The next generation of adjuvant trials may demonstrate that the combination of chemo-endocrine treatments is the "gold standard" in the adjuvant treatment of breast cancer. However, there is a need for considerably more national and international collaboration to obtain maximum information on the combination, duration, and timing of combined treatment modalities.

REFERENCES

1 Paridaens RJ and Piccart MJ: Chemo-hormonal treatment of breast cancer: The state of the art. In: Sluyser M (ed) Growth Factors and Oncogenes in Breast Cancer. Health Sciences Series, Ellis Horwood 1987 pp 193-206

2 Henderson IC: Endocrine therapy of metastatic breast cancer. In: Harris JR, Hellman S, Henderson IC and Kinne DW (eds) Breast Diseases. JB Lippincott Comp, Philadelphia 1991 pp 559-603

3 Henderson IC: Chemotherapy for metastatic disease. In: Harris JR, Hellman S, Henderson IC and Kinne DW (eds) Breast Diseases. JB Lippincott Comp, Philadelphia 1991 pp 604-665

4 Goldhirsch A, Gelber RD, Castiglione M, for the International Breast Cancer Study Group: Adjuvant therapy of breast cancer. Eur J Cancer 1991 (27):389-399

5 Early Breast Cancer Trialists' Collaborative Group: Systemic treatment of early breast cancer by hormonal, cytotoxic, or immune therapy: 133 randomized trials involving 31,000 recurrences and 24,000 deaths among 75,000 women. Lancet 1992 (339):1-15, 71-85

6 Bonadonna G: Evolving concepts in the systemic adjuvant treatment of breast cancer. Cancer Res 1992 (52):2127-2137

7 Fisher B, Wickerham DL, Redmond C: Recent developments in the news of systemic adjuvant therapy for the treatment of breast cancer. Sem Oncol 1992 (19):263-277

8 Goldenberg GJ, Froese EK: Antagonism of the cytocidal activity and uptake of melphalan by tamoxifen in human breast cancer cells in vitro. Biochem Pharmacol 1985 (34):763-770

9 Osborne CK, Kitten L, Antega CL: Antagonism of chemotherapy-induced cytotoxicity for human breast cancer cells by antiestrogens. J Clin Oncol 1989 (7):710-717

10 Kaufmann M, Jonat W, Kleeberg U et al: Goserelin, a depot gonadotrophin-releasing hormone agonist in the treatment of premenopausal patients with metastatic breast cancer. J Clin Oncol 1989 (7):1113-1119

11 Love RR, Mazess RB, Tormey DC, Barden HS, Newcomb PA, Jordan VC: Bone mineral density in women with breast cancer treated with adjuvant tamoxifen for at least two years. Breast Cancer Res Treat 1988 (12):297-302

12 Bruning PF, Bonfrer JM, Hart AA, deJong-Bakker M, Linders D, van Loon J, Nooyen WJ: Tamoxifen, serum lipoproteins and cardiovascular risk. Br J Cancer 1989 (58):497-499

13 Glick JH, Gelber RD, Goldhirsch A, Senn HJ: Meeting highlights: Adjuvant therapy for primary breast cancer. JNCI 1992 (84):1479-1485

14 Rubens RD: Management of early breast cancer. Br Med J 1992 (304):1361-1364

15 Davidson NE, Abeloff MD: Adjuvant systemic therapy in women with early stage breast cancer at high risk for relapse. JNCI 1992 (84):301-304

Quality of Life Measures as Endpoints and Prognostic Factors in Advanced Breast Cancer

Alan S. Coates

Australian New Zealand Breast Cancer Trials Group, Department of Medical Oncology, Royal Prince Alfred Hospital, Camperdown, NSW 2050, Australia

Quality of life (QL) is probably beyond ultimate definition [1], yet we are all conscious that it may vary from time to time and from person to person. It is a common part of human nature to be more aware of the deficiencies that detract from QL rather than of its more positive aspects. In the setting of malignant disease, the physical symptoms, the psychological and social effects of the disease, and the side-effects of its treatment all clearly diminish QL. Decisions made about treatment may improve one symptom, but perhaps at the cost of causing or exacerbating another. Measurement of those aspects of QL related to the manifestations of the disease and the adverse effects of its treatment might therefore be of value in assessing the progress of a particular patient in order to choose the optimal time to change treatment, or in the setting of a clinical trial to compare the average results of different treatment policies so as to guide clinicians to choose programmes which are more likely to lead to a net improvement of QL.

Measurement of QL

Practical tools for the measurement of aspects of QL in the clinical setting are now readily available, although they vary in scope, in complexity, and in the degree to which their validity and reliability have been established. The question may arise as to whether such measurements are sufficiently established and sufficiently scientific to be useful in the understanding or the treatment of breast cancer. It is the purpose of this chapter to show evidence that they are so established: that they outperform many of the traditional endpoints in clinical trials, and that therefore their use, both as endpoints by which treatments may be compared and as prognostic factors by which survival may be predicted, can no longer be ignored.

An important concept in the measurement of QL is the scope of the instruments used - exactly which aspects relevant to QL should be measured, and how should the questions be phrased. Technically, this refers to the concept of variability. A measure which returns essentially identical values for all subjects in a group is of no value in discriminating among them. This in turn requires that the questionnaire should reflect the target population. The magnitude and type of differences in QL among a group of healthy young adults at a holiday resort may have little in common with the variations in a group of patients in a palliative care hospice. The measurement of aspects of QL must therefore be determined by whether the instrument is to be used for all diseases, just for cancers, for a specific cancer, a particular stage of disease, or indeed for a specific therapy trial. In general, some global aspects and some specific aspects of QL will usually be of interest. Thus, the European Organization for Research and Treatment of Cancer (EORTC) QL group uses a core questionnaire across many different cancer trials, but adds specific modules to address aspects of particular interest in a given setting [2]. There is general agreement that patients should assess their own QL, although assessment by the physician is also established as valid and useful [3]. The techniques used for patient self-assess-

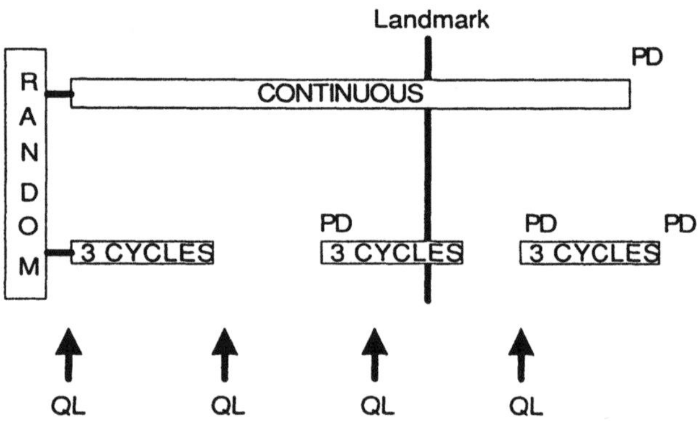

Fig. 1. Continuous versus intermittent cytotoxic chemotherapy in the treatment of metastatic breast cancer: a trial of the Australian New Zealand Breast Cancer Trials Group (ANZ 8101). Intermittent therapy policy consisted of blocks of 3 cycles, either of cyclophosphamide, methotrexate, fluorouracil and prednisone (CMFP) or doxorubicin and cyclophosphamide (DC). PD denotes progressive disease.

ment of QL have included various visual analogue systems [4-8], categorical scales [2], and more complex questionnaires, though there is evidence that all these methods, including particularly the simple, practical self-administered scales, yield similarly useful information [9].

QL as an Endpoint in Clinical Trials

Probably the first investigators to apply QL measurements as endpoints to assist in comparison of various treatments for breast cancer were Priestman et al. These authors initially used a series of 10 linear analogue self-assessment (LASA) scales to monitor subjective benefits of treatment [5], and later expanded the instrument to compare endocrine and cytotoxic treatments for breast cancer [10]. They concluded that effective antitumour therapy improved QL of patients with metastatic breast cancer, and that the induction of objective tumour response, rather than the modality used to achieve the response, was crucial to the improvement in QL. The Australian New Zealand Breast Cancer Trials Group later conducted a clinical trial to compare endocrine, cytotoxic and combined chemo-endocrine therapies for metastatic breast cancer. The results indicated that the initial use of endocrine therapy for metastatic breast cancer was safe, and was not associated with inferior survival in any defined group of patients [11]. Implicit in this study was the belief that controlling disease while delaying the introduction of cytotoxic therapy would confer improved QL, but no explicit QL measurements were included in the trial.

A subsequent study from the Australian New Zealand Breast Cancer Trials Group was directly designed to evaluate QL in the treatment of metastatic breast cancer [12]. The basic question asked was whether intermittent therapy might provide a better cost-benefit balance than the traditional continuous approach (Fig. 1). Continuous and intermittent therapy policies were compared, each using two different chemotherapy combinations. Doxorubicin plus cyclophosphamide (DC) comprised doxorubicin 50 mg/m^2 and cyclophosphamide 750 mg/m^2 intravenously each 21 days. Cyclophosphamide, methotrexate, 5-fluorouracil and prednisone (CMFP) therapy consisted of 28-day cycles with oral cyclophosphamide 100 mg/m^2 and oral prednisone 40 mg/m^2 daily for 14 days, with intravenous methotrexate 40 mg/m^2 and 5-fluorouracil 600 mg/m^2 on days 1 and 8. Patients allocated continuous therapy continued cyclical treatment until disease progression, while those allocated intermittent therapy were observed without treatment after 3 cycles until disease progression, when the same therapy was reintroduced for a further 3 cycles. In addition to the traditional clinical trial endpoints of tumour response rate, time to treatment failure, toxicity scales and overall survival, the trial endpoints included several indicators of QL. Spitzer's QL Index [3] was measured by the doctor. This concise instrument assesses 5 aspects relevant to QL: activity level, daily living, general health, support by others and outlook. Each aspect is scored on a 3-point scale, and the total of the 5 scores forms the Index. All other QL assessments were made by the patients themselves. LASA lines measuring physical well-being (PWB), mood, pain nausea/vomiting (N&V) and appetite were chosen from the scales of Priestman et al. [10]. In addition, the patient completed a single LASA line (uniscale) designed by Spitzer [3] to measure overall QL.

Changes in QL scores during the first 3 treatment cycles, while all patients were receiving therapy, reflected the impact of chemotherapy on QL. As expected, scores for N&V showed deterioration, but those for all other QL endpoints improved during this initial treatment [12]. In the groups allocated intermittent therapy, QL deteriorated after therapy cessation, whereas there was continued improvement among patients continuing therapy. Patient self-assessment of PWB, mood, appetite and uniscale, and physician assessment of QL index showed significant differences in favour of continuous therapy. No difference was detected in the impact of the two chemotherapy combinations on QL, except that patient scores for N&V were worse with DC than with CMFP. The result of this trial showed that QL could be measured in a multi-institutional setting, and could give coherent results. That the results were clearly opposite to the hope which inspired the trial may add some further credibility. Incidentally, the relationship between objective tumour response category and QL in this trial confirmed one of the findings of Priestman et al. [10], in that improvement in QL during the first 3 treatment cycles was seen in patients who achieved a partial or complete objective tumour response, but not in those whose tumours remained stable. Nevertheless, continuous therapy yielded better QL than intermittent therapy even among those with stable disease, indicating that a discernibly useful degree of tumour control was achieved in these patients.

A similar study of less versus more cytotoxic therapy for metastatic breast cancer was conducted at about the same time by Tannock et al. [13], who found that reduced doses of chemotherapy were associated with inferior objective results, and inferior QL as measured by a battery of LASA scales [8]. Taken together, these trials provide powerful evidence that appropriate cytotoxic therapy is worthwhile in advanced breast cancer, in that it improves overall QL because its beneficial effect in terms of tumour control outweighs the side-effects of therapy. This of course reflects carefully monitored treatment in major institutions, and in particular the requirement of both trials that therapy be discontinued when it was no longer effective.

QL as a Prognostic Indicator

The other main value of QL measurements is that they have been shown in studies in breast cancer, lung cancer and melanoma to be powerful and sensitive predictors of subsequent survival duration. In the trial comparing intermittent and continuous therapy policies described above, scores for many of the QL indicators were found to be independent prognostic factors for survival. Physician assessment of the QL index and patient LASA scores for PWB, mood, N&V, appetite and uniscale (but not pain) at the commencement of treatment were significant predictors of subsequent survival. Scores for PWB and QL index remained independently significant even when allowance was made for other prognostic factors (liver metastases, performance status, brain metastases, node metastases and intermittent therapy policy). Serial changes in QL scores were also prognostically important. Both baseline and change in scores for PWB, mood, pain and QL index after the first 3 cycles but before an arbitrary 180-day "landmark" time point were significantly predictive of survival beyond that landmark. The change in scores for mood, pain and QL index were independent of other recorded prognostic factors, and both QL index and PWB scores were prognostically significant even after allowing for objective tumour response [14].

Evidence from Other Tumour Types

The Lung Cancer Study Group found QL as measured by the Functional Living Index - Cancer (FLIC) [7] to be an important prognostic factor in patients undergoing surgery for bronchogenic carcinoma [15], and similar findings were reported by Ganz et al. [16]. In metastatic melanoma, Thomson et al. conducted a trial to test the addition of interferon to dacarbazine chemotherapy [17]. In addition to the QL endpoints described for the Australian New Zealand Breast Cancer Trials Group studies, this trial incorporated a new LASA instrument known as GLQ-8, developed to measure the toxicity of chemotherapy [18]. In this trial, Spitzer's QL Index assessed by the doctor and LASA scores for PWB, mood, pain, appetite, N&V, uniscale and GLQ-8 were all significant predictors of subsequent survival. QL Index and LASA scales for mood, appetite, and uniscale remained independently significant in multivariate models allowing for the other significant prognostic factors (liver metastases and performance status).

These findings, in a variety of tumour types, add to the evidence for validity of the various QL measures used in the trials. They are compatible with the simple explanation that patients perceive disease progression before it is clinically evident to their doctors. If this were all, the measurements would still be of clinical value. However, the data are also compatible with a causal relationship between aspects of quality of life and survival duration. If this were true, it might offer scope for intervention aimed at prolonging survival by improving QL.

Conclusion

QL can be adequately measured by simple, practical methods, and the results provide a useful endpoint by which to judge the net relative cost-benefit values of more and less toxic therapies for advanced cancer. As a bonus, QL measurement provides powerful prognostic information. These findings establish a strong case for the routine measurement of aspects of QL in clinical trials, and the incorporation of formal QL evaluation as part of everyday clinical oncology practice.

REFERENCES

1 Aaronson NK, Meyerowitz BE, Bard M, Bloom JR, Fawzy FI, Feldstein M, Fink D, Holland JC, Johnson JE, Lowman JT, Patterson WB and Ware JE: Quality of life research in oncology. Past achievements and future priorities. Cancer 1991 (67):839-843

2 Aaronson NK, Bullinger M and Ahmedzai S: A modular approach to quality of life assessment in cancer clinical trials. Recent Results in Cancer Research 1988 (111): 231-249

3 Spitzer WO, Dobson AJ, Hall J, Chesterman E, Levi J, Shepherd R, Battista RN and Catchlove BR: Measuring the quality of life of cancer patients: a concise QL index for use by physicians. J Chron Dis 1981 (34):585-597

4 Aitken RCB: Measurement of feelings using visual analogue scales. Proc Royal Soc Med 1969 (62): 989-996

5 Priestman TJ, Baum M: Evaluation of quality of life in patients receiving treatment for advanced breast cancer. Lancet 1976 (1):899-901

6 Coates AS, Fischer Dillenbeck C, McNeil DR, Kaye SB, Sims K, Fox RM, Hedley D, Raghavan D, Woods RL, Milton GW and Tattersall MHN: On the receiving end - II. Linear analog self assessment (LASA) in evaluation of aspects of the quality of life of cancer patients receiving therapy. Eur J Cancer Clin Oncol 1983 (19):1633-1637

7 Schipper H, Clinch J, McMurray A, Levitt M: Measuring the quality of life of cancer patients: the functional living index - cancer: development and validation. J Clin Oncol 1984 (2):472-483

8 Selby P, Robertson B: Measurement of quality of life in patients with cancer. Cancer Surveys 1987 (6):521-543

9 Butow P, Coates AS, McNeil DR, Dunn S: On the receiving end IV: validation of quality of life instruments. Ann Oncol 1991 (2):597-603

10 Priestman T, Baum M, Jones V, Forbes J: Comparative trial of endocrine versus cytotoxic treatment in advanced breast cancer. Br Med J 1977 (1):1248-1250

11 Australia-New Zealand Breast Cancer Trials Group: A randomized trial in postmenopausal patients with advanced breast cancer comparing endocrine and cytotoxic therapy given sequentially or in combination. J Clin Oncol 1986 (4):186-193

12 Coates A, Gebski V, Bishop JF, Jeal PN, Woods RL, Snyder R, Tattersall MHN, Byrne M, Harvey V, Gill G, Simpson J, Drummond R, Browne J, Van Cooten R and Forbes JF for the ANZ Breast Cancer Trials Group: Improving the quality of life during chemotherapy for advanced breast cancer. A comparison of intermittent and continuous treatment strategies. N Engl J Med 1987 (317):1490-1495

13 Tannock IF, Boyd N, De Boer G, Erlichman C, Fine S, Larocque G, Mayers C, Perrault D and Sutherland S: A randomized trial of two dose levels of cyclophosphamide, methotrexate and fluorouracil chemotherapy for patients with metastatic breast cancer. J Clin Oncol 1988 (6):1377-1387

14 Coates AS, Gebski V, Signorini D, Murray P, McNeil DR, Byrne M and Forbes JF for the Australian New Zealand Breast Cancer Trials Group: Prognostic value of quality of life scores during chemotherapy for advanced breast cancer. J Clin Oncol 1992 (10):1833-1838

15 Ruckdeschel JC, Piantadosi S and the Lung Cancer Study Group: Quality of life assessment in lung surgery for bronchogenic carcinoma. Theoret Surg 1991 (6):201-205

16 Ganz PA, Lee JJ and Siau J: Quality of life assessment. An independent prognostic variable for survival in lung cancer. Cancer 1991 (67):3131-3135

17 Thomson D, Adena M, Hersey P, Gill PG, Coates AS, Olver IN, Kefford R, Lowenthal R, Beadle G, Walpole E, Boland K and Kingston D: Interferon alpha-2a does not improve response or survival when added to dacarbazine in metastatic melanoma: results of a multi-institutional Australian randomized trial QMP8704. Proc Amer Soc Clin Oncol 1992 (11):343 (#1177)

18 Coates AS, Glasziou P and McNeil DR: On the receiving end III: measurement of quality of life during cancer chemotherapy. Ann Onc 1990 (1):213-217

19 Coates AS, Thomson D, McLeod GRM, Hersey P, Gill PG, Olver IN, Kefford R, Lowenthal RM, Beadle G and Walpole E: Prognostic value of quality of life scores in a trial of chemotherapy with or without interferon in patients with metastatic malignant melanoma. Eur J Cancer 1993 (in press)

MIX
Papier aus verantwortungsvollen Quellen
Paper from responsible sources
FSC® C105338

If you have any concerns about our products,
you can contact us on
ProductSafety@springernature.com

In case Publisher is established outside the EU,
the EU authorized representative is:
Springer Nature Customer Service Center GmbH
Europaplatz 3, 69115 Heidelberg, Germany

Printed by Libri Plureos GmbH
in Hamburg, Germany